"Bill Hansen has outlined a lifestyle that has proven results to beat Parkinson's, and most importantly, he gives all the tools and background information to help the reader follow his path."
— Lisa Tataryn, B.Sc.R.P.C.C.N.P.,
Center for Neurofeedback and
Research

"I am astonished at how quickly I responded to all of Bill Hansen's products. My mind and body feel extremely stable. I can't remember the last time I got out of bed so many days in a row looking forward to tackle my day."
— Beverly Hall

"Several years ago, Bill Hansen looked terrible, his hands shook so badly, he was pathetically thin, and he'd taken on a "mask-like" expression. After one and one-half years, his recovery was a miracle. The products he produces and his spirituality is what gave him back his life and his health."
— B. Adams, San Marcos, CA

" . . . I have nothing but praise to share with you regarding your product and how meaningful my physical and emotional response has been . . . I am experiencing clarity of mind and thought . . . and my speech is, for the most part, clear and without a slur. Thank you, Bill, and God Bless."
— Lorraine Butler

Visit our Web site: www.noparkinsons.net

"I have been training Bill for a year and a half and have been completely amazed by his improvements. The fact that Bill has Parkinson's made me question how his training would go. With Bill's consistent workouts and spray nutritionals (BODY), positive attitude (MIND), and his early morning quiet time (SPIRIT), he has far exceeded my expectations."

— Heather Young, AFFA, Trainer
Fitness/Counselor.

"Bill does not claim to have found a "cure" for Parkinson's but from what I have seen with my own eyes, the hope his oral sprays offer will seem like nothing less than a miracle to those who currently have none. I am grateful to know this man, and the passion with which he has dedicated his life to alleviating the suffering of others."

— Reverend Nancy Berggren,
Senior Minister, Church of
Religious Science

"Your book offers more than hope. You provide a roadmap of things to do, things to read, and a way of living that would serve to improve anyone's life."

— Lael Jackson-Actress

"I can easily see how reading this book could help anyone with any physical problems, especially someone who is already on your wave length. Thanks for this chance to become inspired."

— Betty Ritter-Author

I'm Dancing Again Because

Hope Heals

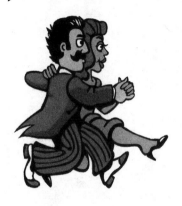

How One Man
Conquered Parkinson's

I'm Dancing Again Because

Hope Heals

How One Man
Conquered Parkinson's

William Paul Hansen, R.C.L.

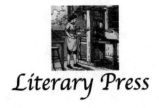

Literary Press

Newport Beach, California
www.literarypress.com

Literary Press
3857 Birch St. Suite 702
Newport Beach, CA 92660
800-339-0551
www.literarypress.com

Library of Congress Control No. 2004103648
ISBN 0-9716958-5-7

Parkimin™ is a registered trademark of MJB Global, Inc.

Cover and interior design by Sparrow Advertising & Design

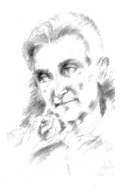

Dedication

This book is dedicated to the readers who will find the spirit of wellness within. May you dance and run again when you realize that *Hope Heals*.

Acknowledgements

The list of people I would like to acknowledge, who made this project possible, would fill another book, so sadly, I can't thank them all by name. All of you know who you are, and I will be eternally grateful for your untiring efforts.

I wish to thank everyone in my family, going all the way back to the genesis into the health and the spray nutraceuticals, who gave of their time and money to assist with this book.

Heartfelt thanks go out to my good friend Webb Lowe, who introduced me to the spray concept, and to Leigh Carrol who had amazing organizing agility, and a most generous nature, and then went on to become one of our first stockholders.

During the Parkimin era, Donna McCollum, who represents all that is good in a person, exhibited a faith in the Parkimin project that can only be exceeded by her grace and her dedication to serve the world.

Other sacred contracts that will never be forgotten are John Prieskorn, Nancy Berggren and Esther Jones.

And finally, last but not least, Robert Bruce Woodcox. Here's a man who goes above and beyond the call of duty. From good writing with an unusual flair for capturing the spirit of the project, to giving guidance in the business of publishing as well. When I was lacking, his poetic license and strength brought my book to reality through the spirit.

A Letter to the Reader from the Publisher

This book has the potential to end a great deal of suffering in this world, and save thousands of lives. That is why I published it. If you have Parkinson's or know someone who does, you may at first be skeptical, but I urge you to read this with an open mind, for William Hansen's story doesn't come from a neurologist's files, it comes from his heart and from thousands of hours of research and experimentation. He was his own guinea pig.

His miraculous story is one of struggle and triumph. It is the inspiring account of the amazing things that can happen when an individual combines the power of a united Spirit, Mind and Body. Ultimately, and above all else, it is a story of hope for every person who suffers not only from Parkinson's, but from any of the neurological disorders such as Alzheimer's, ALS, MS, and others. Let me introduce him to you. . . .

I first met Bill in his home in Carlsbad, California, in September of 2003. He had obtained my name from the Internet. When he first told me his story briefly over the phone several weeks prior to our meeting, I am now ashamed to say, I didn't believe him. According to him, he had developed a regimen, which included some new neutraceutical sprays—vitamin and amino acid combinations, which his company had manufactured. These, in combination with an effective protocol, had alleviated 90 percent of his Parkinson's symptoms.

"No, I wasn't cured but yes, I could dance again," he said.

At the time, I knew next to nothing about the disease, so I told him I would conduct some research of my own and get back to him. After reading a couple of books and visiting various Web sites, I learned just how devastating the disease is; how those who are afflicted, usually in their sixties and seventies, all but shrivel up and eventually die. I read how these people lost nearly all control of their motor functions, including the ability to swallow. As the disease progresses from simple tremors in the beginning to a point where a person cannot walk, or even roll over in bed, it renders its victims completely helpless.

It saddened me deeply to realize that more than 1 million people are afflicted, and more than 50,000 people contract it each year. In the beginning, symptoms range from mild tremors of the hands to an increasingly weakened and debilitated state. Facial muscles (Parkinson's Mask) don't move; the patient has great difficulty swallowing some types of food. They develop cramps; loss of appetite; and in some cases, severe weight loss; and eventually the afflicted cannot even move without help. Later, this can lead to hospitalization or hospice where the patient must be fed intravenously and cleaned up after by a nurse, attendant, or family member.

Not only does the disease rob the victim of his or her motor skills, it steals his or her dignity slowly and insidiously until many patients also fall into a deep depression.

The final stage is death.

I learned what causes the disease and how it is treated. There are several drugs currently being used. However, drug treatments are only temporary and only slightly effective on a day-by-day or week-by-week basis. There is also a surgical procedure that is used with limited success.

Mainstream medicine has no solution and no cure. Patients are most often given the drug therapy and then told to do the best they can. The diagnosis is usually the same. You will get worse and eventually die. In the meantime, we can try to make you as comfortable as possible, which of course, is no comfort at all.

In short, no doctor or patient has ever reported, in any mainstream publication or other media, that a treatment has been found to effectively eliminate all of the symptoms of the disease.

At this point, I had to admit I was interested in speaking with Mr. Hansen. I had to see firsthand if he was a quack or not. He had told me he was seventy-four and that he'd had the disease for six and a half years. If that were true, he would surely be quite feeble and almost certainly not ambulatory to any significant degree. We made an appointment to meet at 2:00 P.M. on September 16, 2003, at his home in Carlsbad. I arrived on time and rang the doorbell. Within seconds, a bright-eyed man, who looked about fifty, answered the door, beaming a broad smile at me and offering his hand. He said, "Hello, Robert. I'm so glad you could come."

He motioned for me to come into his bright, neatly arranged living room. Again, he smiled and said, "Have a seat. Take a load off."

I had to admit; I was stunned and pleasantly surprised to see him walk quickly and effortlessly to the kitchen to bring me a glass of water. When he returned, he said, as he began to twirl in circles, "I'm dancin' again."

I had no idea what he was talking about, though he did appear to be doing some vigorous jitterbug steps.

"I don't know how much you know about Parkinson's," he said, "but I can tell you that, to my knowledge, there are few others in the advanced stages of this disease who walk with any confidence, let alone dance like me."

By now, Mr. Hansen was practically doing cartwheels in his glee to demonstrate his abilities. Finally, he bounced into a chair next to me and began to talk. Within a few minutes, he was showing me a videotape, which had once aired on CNN, showing Parkinson's patients working with a neurologist. Each patient depicted had been told by the doctor to walk back and forth in a hallway with the assistance of a nurse. The footage was difficult to watch. These poor people wore what Bill would later tell me was "The

Parkinson's Mask," something he'd worn as well. The mask is marked by a lack of any emotion, though the people on the tape looked quite sad.

The first patient looked as if his feet were nailed to the floor. He apparently was trying to accomplish a 180-degree turn, but despite the best efforts of his mind to convince his legs to move, they would not. Neither would his arms. Each effort to even put one foot in front of the other appeared to be a monumental undertaking.

After these patients were given injections of an amino acid called glutathione, a natural brain antioxidant, the results were astounding. Not thirty minutes after the injections, they were smiling brightly, swinging their arms, and striding quickly back and forth down the hall.

I had read some information about these injections and, as it turns out, it is one of two effective substances on the market today (by effective, it offers temporary relief). The other substance is Sinamet, the current gold standard for treatment in a pill form.

"Pretty remarkable, huh?" Bill said. "Only problem is, the effects of those injections only last a day or two at most, and they cost close to $100 each. The patient gets a big high right away and then it quickly diminishes. It's like a roller coaster ride. They have to come back three, four, or even five times a week to keep the effect going. Would you call that a viable alternative?"

"No. Not many people could afford $500 a week in treatments and my guess is not many HMOs would pay for it," I replied.

"You're a bright young man," Bill said, as he flashed another big smile, revealing a set of perfectly straight, white teeth. At that moment, I took a closer and longer look at his face. He'd told me he was seventy-four, but he didn't look a day over fifty-five. He had brilliant blue eyes, with perhaps a wrinkle or two around the edges, but his skin was clear and smooth and he had a full head of hair. In short, he looked far healthier than most of my friends who are in their late forties and early fifties.

"You know, it's not just the sprays I use that erase the symptoms. It's really a combination of the Spirit, Mind and Body acting in concert. The body part includes exercise and diet, though the diet I'm on is a simple mainstream regimen, and it's only the icing on the cake, as far as I'm concerned. I attribute most of my recovery to the sprays, my spiritual beliefs, and a consistent exercise program."

"Okay, wait a minute Bill. Let's sit down and start at the beginning. What sprays? What kind of exercise?" I asked.

"It's the combination of bringing together the Spirit, Mind, and Body—but, of course, the real engine is the sprays we've created. Even if someone didn't do the workouts I do or use the same diet, he could still see a marked reduction in his (or her) symptoms just by using the sprays on a daily basis. It's just that the program works much faster and more effectively when your life is in complete balance.

"Here, read this," he said as he handed me a slip of paper on which was typed neatly this message:

Guidance . . .

When I meditate on the word guidance, I keep seeing "dance" at the end of the word. I remember reading that God's Will is a lot like dancing.

When two people try to lead, nothing feels right. The movement doesn't flow with the music, and everything is quite uncomfortable and jerky. When one person relaxes and lets the other lead, both bodies begin to flow with the music. One gives gentle cues, perhaps with a nudge to the back or by pressing lightly in one direction or another.

It's as if two become one body, moving beautifully in sync. The dance takes surrender, willingness, and attentiveness from one person and gentle guidance and skill from the other.

When I saw the "G," in guidance, I thought of God, followed by the "u" and the "i". "God"—"u" and "i" dance.

That's what guidance means to me. As I lower my head, I become willing to trust that I will get guidance about my life. I will let go and let God.

I had to admit I was utterly enthralled with this energetic man with the inviting smile and engaging attitude. I wanted to know more. In those hours, and many more that followed over the next three months, William Hansen told me his story.

His ordeal began in June of 1997 and ended in the fall of 2001. At the three and a half year mark of his disease, he was deteriorating rapidly. His daily regimen was severely restricted and he could not even turn over in bed without great effort. Unless he took pains to eat extremely slowly, he would have great difficulty chewing foods like chicken, or beef and would often have to stick his finger down his throat to regurgitate. This usually happened in public when he was out with friends and did not pay attention to how fast he was eating (of course, he would always have to excuse himself and rush to the restroom).

At the five-year mark, having single-handedly created his own very successful treatment protocol (he stopped taking the advice of his neurologist, with the exception of the use of Sinamet), he is truly "dancin' again."

Though challenged from time to time, Bill Hansen is thriving physically, mentally, and spiritually. He is the picture of health and fulfillment and wears a perpetual smile, and he dances three nights a week in local clubs and restaurants. He loves to jitterbug, but his favorite is the cha-cha, something he couldn't do until a year ago.

In addition, his physical regimen includes time on the stationary bicycle, treadmill, and free weights, which he does three times a week.

Here is William Hansen's remarkable true story. It is the story of the evolution of a seeker. It is his wish that if you have Parkinson's, or know someone who does, you will use this information to help set yourself and others free from the ravages of this disease. He asks that you help spread the word to as many people as you can. When you're through reading this book, give it to a friend who might need your help or, better yet, *buy* two more and give them away.

A significant portion of the proceeds of this book goes to fight Parkinson's and other neurological disorders through the following organizations: From the MJB Global, Inc. (Nutraceuticals), 10 percent of revenues go to children's charities. From the sale of this book, (Parkimin Technologies) 15 percent of the proceeds go to alternative medicine or complimentary medicine research and studies.

Bill Hansen wants you to know that the writing of this book was a labor of great love for his fellow man, particularly those who have been stricken with Parkinson's or any other neurological disorder. He knew the best way to tell his story, in order to help others, would be to write a bestseller.

For the past three years, Bill's passion and purpose has been to get this information out to others so that they could experience the same delicious freedom he has.

> Robert Bruce Woodcox
> Publisher
> Literary Press

At about the same time Bill was diagnosed with Parkinson's, he was also found to have prostate cancer. At one point about a year prior to the writing of this book, his PSA level was an astounding 155 (normal is about 4.0). Today, as we finish this book, he was retested and his PSA level was 3.5.

I stand on the shoulders of my past.
I know and accept that I am who I am
because of my past experiences.
I cannot deny that they are
a huge part of who I am today.
My past is my history
and I choose to accept it all
as part of my spiritual and personal growth—
therefore, <u>it is all good.</u>
Who I am is the sum total of everything that
I have thought, learned, and experienced.
I choose to honor and respect every area of my life
and every person and experience
that has contributed to my life.

With heartfelt thanks to my dear friend, Esther Jones.

Chapter One

I was floating that night, feeling on top of the world. Several months prior, Sandi had accepted my marriage proposal and tonight she sat at my side at the dinner table. I quietly rehearsed the speech I was about to give to the class of 1947, reading to her from my notes.

It was my fiftieth high school reunion and sixty of us were seated in the ballroom at the beautiful Hotel Del Coronado near San Diego.

Tables were covered in starched white linen cloths, each with an enormous flower arrangement. The place settings were ornate bone china complimented by crystal wine glasses.

Though I was excited about seeing my dear friends, I was also nervous about speaking to so many people.

It was in June of 1997 and I will never forget the evening if I live to be a hundred. Though I didn't know it at the time, I would experience the very first symptoms of Parkinson's disease in front of my soon-to-be bride and all my high school friends.

Just then the master of ceremonies, who had finished introducing me, was asking me to come up to the podium.

When I reached the dais, he handed me the microphone, shook my hand, and walked down the stairs. I cleared my throat and reminded myself to thank everyone for attending. As I brought the mike up to my mouth, my hand began to shake violently and uncontrollably. It must have been obvious to everyone in the room, though no one said anything. Quickly shifting the microphone to my left hand, my first thought was that I had a case of stage fright. *However, if that were the case, why was my left hand steady?*

As I regained my composure and began to talk, I placed my still-trembling right hand on the podium to keep it from jerking about. It felt like an alien appendage, like watching a fish flopping about on dry land.

Somehow I managed to get through my presentation as Sandi smiled at me from the dinner table. I should have been quite happy. Instead, I was scared. I knew something was wrong with me, something terribly wrong.

All my life I had been athletic, involved in track and field in high school. I was also a young lifeguard on Del Mar beach in the summertime and played football in college. I couldn't remember a day that I was sick, other than a bout with a cold once in awhile. Even with all those sports, I was never seriously injured; I suppose I never thought about it, but subconsciously, I felt invincible. However, now that I was sixty-eight, it appeared my luck was running out.

"Essential tremors. Nothing serious really. I have some medicine I'm going to prescribe that will help control them. Other than that, you're fine," the doctor blithely said, and I accepted his diagnosis; after all, he was a respected physician. I believed him.

The pills did not help and over the next two years I slowly, but progressively got worse. At first, my balance was off and eventually my coordination suffered greatly, and I found myself clumsily stumbling into, or dropping things. My loss of appetite was less noticeable to me, but it became quite apparent when my family realized I'd lost about fifteen pounds. Compounding my loss of appetite was my difficulty swallowing when I *did* want to eat, especially chicken or beef. Eventually, I would have to go to the bathroom and force myself to regurgitate the partially chewed food.

At my worst, I could barely even turn over in bed, a maneuver that required a complete force of will. In my mind, I knew I wanted to turn over, but my body would not respond. It was as if the lines of communication were disconnecting—and indeed they were. As I would ultimately discover.

At times, it was a great effort just to walk around the house. I would find myself standing at the kitchen sink, the doorbell would ring, and the natural instincts in my mind would say, *"Go answer the door,"* but my legs would not move. After awhile, I would have to use an enormous amount of will power to turn my body and put one leg in front of the other. I would have to say, *Bill, extend your right leg, now your left,* and so on until perhaps a few minutes later I would arrive at the door. On some occasions, the visitor had left before I could get there.

When I was finally diagnosed with Parkinson's after seeing several different doctors, they simply said it was incurable, that the symptoms would continue to get worse, and that my only option was to learn to live with it. In the end, it would kill me, they said. This time I didn't accept their diagnosis. A mild tremor was one thing, Parkinson's was another. People often ask me if I was scared or angry, the most common reactions to life threatening illnesses. I have to answer them honestly and tell them no. As you get to know me throughout this book, you'll come to understand why I wasn't afraid. For now, however, I can tell you that my strongest reaction was embarrassment, even humiliation—not because I had contracted the disease, but because my movements were

WHAT IS THE OPPOSITE OF LOVE? NO, IT ISN'T HATE; IT'S FEAR AND IT'S MANIFESTED THROUGH EGO.

so inhibited. My tremors embarrassed me a great deal, so much so that when I was with people, if my hands began to shake, I would sit on them. I also had great trouble writing. The simplest note was an agonizing undertaking—the sentences barely legible, a scrawl across the page. This was particularly embarrassing if I had to write something in front of someone.

Eventually, trying to hide my tremors and all the other symptoms just became a living lie. I was hiding what I believed at the time to be my weaknesses. I felt this disease was my fault. It got so that I had to carefully plan every minute of every day to accommodate my *problem* by trying to conceal my tremors and poor motor skills—a terrible emotional burden. I was filled with guilt and humiliation.

I would wait until the afternoons to make any phone calls, until my voice had some semblance of strength. For some reason, I usually felt a little better in the afternoons than I did in the mornings, so anyone I had to meet with was scheduled later in the day.

I was also confused. One of the first things I asked myself was, why have I brought this into my life? You'll also discover the answer to that question within my story.

Having spent most of my life as a seeker, I understand very well the evil that *ego* creates in so many forms; and yet, trying to hide my tremors was just that, a "giving in" to my ego. Like everything else, however, there is always a positive aspect. Though most of us would do well to eliminate many of our emotions from our thinking processes, especially the negative ones, emotions do play a powerful role in causing us to take action, which is exactly what I did.

The emotion of humiliation lit a fire under me, and the first thing I did was to buy as many books and tapes on the subject of Parkinson's as I could find. I was not going to give into it. I was consumed by a passion to learn how to conquer this disease.

I remember lying awake for hours at night devouring the available literature. The only thing that kept me from reading was my tremors. Sometimes I would have to hold the book with one hand and use my other hand to hold onto my wrist to steady myself enough to be able to focus on the words. In the beginning, most of the literature was negative and did not hold out hope. However, that would later change dramatically.

Prior to this point in my life, I was an avid dancer. One of my favorite pastimes was to whirl away the evening with friends dancing. Now, my coordination was failing me. I was deteriorating rapidly and it began to depress me.

Imagine having been involved all your life in sports, loving to jog perhaps, or being an avid skier, or finding joy in dancing, only to suddenly have your legs shot out from under you, so to speak.

Looking back, I guess I can thank the Lord that at least I wasn't confined to a wheelchair. Yet, there were days when all I wanted to do was sit in a chair.

Oftentimes, I didn't even bother to answer the phone, even though I had one near me because my voice had become so weak. Some people could barely hear what I was saying.

In addition to the physical manifestations of the disease, there were the emotional factors to deal with too. I had my bouts with depression, but thankfully, they weren't as bad as some of the cases I had read about (many Parkinson's sufferers regularly contemplate suicide out of severe depression).

In my *mind*, I still felt like the active and vibrant man I'd always been; my body just wouldn't go along with the program. As I read about others with the disease, it bothered me to no end to think about those who ultimately wound up in hospital beds having a nurse or attendant clean up their messes, unable to even move.

In all, the constant tension and anxiety are nearly as debilitating as the physical symptoms. Eventually, it all begins to weigh mightily on your emotional state and most who suffer slowly, day by day, begin to give up. And why not, especially when you are bombarded with messages of hopelessness from the medical establishment.

As you will soon discover in these pages, eventually by shear force of will, born out of frustration and humiliation, I began to take the steps that ultimately led to my recovery. One day at a time, I found a way to have hope (which I feel is the primary factor that contributes to recovery). And I found that hope through a combination of my faith, the positive effects I was experiencing from my nutritional sprays (more on this important factor shortly), and my physical efforts to rehabilitate my strength and coordination. I also know that my competitive spirit was instilled in me by my mother and father, coaches and teachers.

> THE HOPEFUL MAN
> SEES SUCCESS WHERE
> OTHERS SEE FAILURE;
> SUNSHINE WHERE
> OTHERS SEE
> SHADOWS AND
> STORMS.
> —O.S. MARDEN

Because of my background and all the support I've had throughout my life, my initial frustrations and humiliations gave way relatively quickly.

From the outset, I was determined to study this disease, seek my own answers, and cure myself. This inquisitiveness and persistence all but blocked out any fear. It is what gave me hope. Without hope, we are doomed and that is the primary reason I am writing this book—to demonstrate beyond any doubt that *you* have reason to hope. Once you read my story and learn about the astounding things that became a part of my life, you will also be able to set yourself on a path of self-healing.

Hope isn't just being optimistic. Nor is it just an intangible emotion that is difficult to get your arms around. Rather, hope is born out of an unshakable belief that you *will* get better. In fact, as you'll find out as you read on, there is a very scientific and biological basis for this emotion and its astonishing curative powers.

Now, if you'll allow me to digress, it is important that you know a little bit about me in order to understand how I emerged victorious over this insidious disease, and how, if you have Parkinson's, you can too!

Chapter Two

In November of 2003, I was preparing to speak at my mother, Nola's funeral. She was ninety-five when she passed away, bless her soul. I had been trying to decide which of the wonderful stories I would tell about this lovely woman. At the same time, I was making notes on what to include in this book. Suddenly an answer to both questions came to me like the crack of a whip. I would begin my talk about my mother and my book with the same story. . . .

It was 1948. I was about to graduate from high school in Coronado, California. I had been living with my uncle and aunt for ten years, ever since my parents were killed in a horrible automobile accident in Blackfoot, Idaho, in 1938. I was eight years old. Four people were in the car, my parents, my sister, and a friend. My sister Marge, who I called my angel sister, and the friend survived.

Of course, I was devastated when they were killed and felt horribly alone and empty.

I was lucky though. I had become very close to my Aunt Nola and Uncle Grant, and when they took me in, I considered them to be my mother and father.

Those days in Coronado were some of the happiest of my life, and were certainly some of the strongest building experiences. My new parents were the only connective tissue to my heritage, to who I truly was. Though my real parents had often passed along fascinating stories about our family, since they had died, there were many things they weren't able to share with me.

> COURAGE ALLOWS THE SUCCESSFUL WOMAN TO FAIL— AND TO LEARN POWERFUL LESSONS FROM THE FAILURE— SO THAT IN THE END, SHE DIDN'T FAIL AT ALL.
> —MAYA ANGELO

I do, however, vividly remember the astounding story of my great-grandmother Soffe. I come from a long line of Mormons dating back to 1863 when great-grandmother Soffe traveled from Malmu, Sweden to the great plains of America, and eventually landed in Salt Lake City, Utah, site of the Mormon Church.

The fact that she even traveled that far in 1863 at the tender age of only sixteen was interesting, but *how* she got there was a study in deep-seated perseverance and determinism; traits that most of my family share.

Great-grandmother Soffe finally reached the banks of the Iowa River via the train, after arriving in New York on a tramp steamer months before. In those days, the train only went to Iowa City. The group set up temporary camp to rest and during that first night, someone stole her shoes; her only pair.

As Great-grandma Soffe and others set out to complete their journey to Salt Lake, she was the only one walking barefoot.

At first, she managed to find some discarded pieces of cloth, which she used to fashion sock-like protection at least. However, these didn't hold up long under the harsh conditions and soon she was barefoot again.

It is 1,300 miles from the banks of the Iowa River to the Temple Square in Salt Lake City, and dear Great-grandma Soffe walked every inch of it. One entry in her journal read, "My feet are so sore I leave bloody footprints in the sand."

While living in Salt Lake, Great-grandma became the third wife of George Nimrod Soffe, who was twenty-five years her senior. Always the determined one, she actually built a home of adobe with twelve-inch thick walls for their eight children by herself. The house is still standing and one day I am going to buy it.

They had eight children; the fifth child was my grandmother. The last time I saw Great-grandma Soffe was at my parents' funeral in 1938. I remember her last words to me. I was filled with anger that my parents had died, and felt particularly angry at the people who'd caused the terrible accident. She said, "Bill, don't ever get angry. It's as great a sin to take offense as it is to give it." I was eight and I've never forgotten her words or her indomitable spirit.

Life with my new parents
in Southern California

Though I loved my new parents dearly, they were busy people, often away at work. My father was a designer of jigs and fixtures at a company called Consolidated Vultee Aircraft, and my mother was a hard-working manager at a firm called Brentwood Egg Co., both jobs they'd taken on shortly after moving from Idaho to Southern California. Because of my parents' busy schedules, my coaches, teachers, and the parents of my friends became my mentors.

In those days, and for many years afterward in college, athletics were my lifeblood. I thrived on football, track, and field (pole vaulting in particular). And I loved the attention and guidance I received from my coaches and teachers as a result of my dedication to sports. From them, I learned to never give up—never! No matter how difficult the situation, I always knew I would get through it. I always had a sense of hope and resiliency.

It was August of 1945. The war had been over for nearly a year. In the summer between my sophomore and junior years in high school, I had my first job; I was a garbage man on North Island, home to the San Diego Naval Base.

As you might expect, it was mindless work, but I enjoyed the physicality of it. As far as I was concerned, anything that helped me build muscle was a plus that would just increase my endurance for football the following fall.

I worked with several young Hispanic boys shoveling the garbage that the trucks dropped off, into an enormous incinerator. We were given large coal shovels and from the early morning until late afternoon, we scooped and heaved until we could barely lift our arms. It was my first encounter with Hispanic people, on a day-to-day basis. Two of them spoke English, the other two were the children of illegal immigrants who often told me stories about their lives in Tijuana; and though they didn't complain, their descriptions were bleak. Getting to know them that summer gave me a completely new perspective on my life and other people, especially those who didn't have the things I had. It was the first time I realized that everyone has the same kinds of dreams for their futures, and the same disappointments.

Despite the fact that I slung garbage all that summer, I always considered Coronado the greatest blessing for a young boy growing up. The weather was sublime and everyone—from my friends to my coaches, teachers, and my friends' parents—was fantastic to me.

I look back now and realize that these people were my first mentors. They taught me the fundamentals of a principled life. I must have been blessed early because I can't remember a person that I was involved with who didn't impart strong moral and ethical lessons to me. Or perhaps I just instinctively steered clear of negative people.

The following summer, I moved up quite a few rungs on the employment ladder, by becoming a delivery truck driver for a fine foods store. In the early morning hours,

I would visit the bakeries and fresh produce stands and pick up deliveries for people who would call the store for home delivery.

Between my junior and senior year, during that summer in 1946, I went to the nearby town of Del Mar and got a tremendous job as a beach boy. Part of my responsibilities were to clean up all the seaweed the tide had spewed on the beach in front of the Del Mar Hotel, a fabulous resort, and then to dig a large hole and bury it all before the early morning guests arrived to soak up the sun and the beautiful Southern California weather.

THE BEST PART OF ONE'S LIFE IS THE WORKING PART, THE CREATIVE PART. BELIEVE ME, I LOVE TO SUCCEED. HOWEVER, THE REAL SPIRITUAL AND EMOTIONAL EXCITEMENT IS IN THE DOING.
—GARRISON KANIN

I was given a large heavy pitchfork for the task and being the "jock" that I was, I turned the whole chore into a game—a race, to be exact. I would run all over the edge of the beach where the sand met the surf, stopping at each strand or lump of the large string-bean-like plants, scoop them up with the pitchfork and then run to the next pile. When the fork would hold no more, I made a mad dash for the hole that I had spent half an hour digging that morning at the uppermost part of the beach and pitch it in. I repeated this dig and dash routine for as long as it took to make the beach sparkle, which was generally a couple of hours.

When I returned to school that fall and rejoined my football buddies, I was delightfully surprised to find that I was now the fastest guy on the team; I had shaved nearly six-tenths of a second off my 100 yard dash times, thanks to my summer games. I attributed it to the fact that the sand was so soft, that I had to really high-step it a countless number of times for the nearly thirty yards from the surf to the rocks.

When I graduated later that year, I returned to the beaches I loved in Del Mar and got a job cleaning up around the pool areas. Soon, though, I was promoted to lifeguard assistant. The head guard was a man named Bill Southard, who had the enviable job of giving swimming lessons to the likes of Betty Grable, Victoria James (daughter of the jazz musician, Harry James), and many other notables who came to the famed resort during the summer. Of course, I was thrilled to help.

I was in heaven. I was using my athletic skills, turning a more golden brown with each passing day, meeting movie stars, and making the unheard of salary of $1.00 an hour, plus whatever I earned giving swimming lessons. This was quite a bit more than my garbage-shoveling job, but to be honest, I probably would have done it for nothing.

But, wait, it gets even better!

At night, I would go up on the patio after dinner and dance with all the beautiful rich girls, daughters of the various celebrities and wealthy businesspeople who would sometimes stay at the hotel for weeks at a time.

To this day, that hotel holds fond memories for me. Just the thought of its majestic architecture, location, and the reminiscences of the "good life" can make me feel warm all over. Of course, I never wanted that summer to end so when my mother told me in late June that I had to go to Utah to live with my grandmother, I was devastated. I remember it as if it were yesterday.

"But Mom, I can't go to Utah. I've got a scholarship to play football for El Centro Junior College," I pleaded.

My mother just looked at me thoughtfully, with the twinge of a smile, and finally said, "Don't they play football in Utah?"

Thinking I might not make a big university team, I replied with only a dimwitted, "Well, yeah, but BYU is such a big school."

In her wisdom, however, she knew I would adapt and without a doubt make the team.

That summer I shipped out for Provo, Utah, to live with my grandmother, Dorothy Hansen Cassity, my real father's mother. In the fall, I enrolled at Brigham Young. As my wise mother predicted, I easily made the team, and played football for two years. I also ran and pole-vaulted for the track team in the spring.

The following summer, I moved in with my mother's father, William S. Manson, and my grandmother. He was a coal miner in a town called Kenilworth, and although that was Mormon country, they were not regular Churchgoers—yet they were the kindest, sweetest people you can imagine. They cared for me as if I were their own son.

Moving to Utah

Many people in my family were involved in the Mormon Church, but it wasn't until I began going to BYU that I became seriously involved with the faith. I loved the school, the people, and was fascinated with the Mormon religion.

That first summer, in 1948, between my freshman and sophomore years, my granddad got me a job in the coal mines. It paid the princely sum of $1.73 an hour.

Grandpa Manson was an old Scot and he was frugal with a dollar. He had to be to survive. Therefore, once I started working, my grandmother started charging me room and board, which I gladly paid to help make ends meet. After all, I was eighteen and I ate like a horse, not just because I was young, but also because the work was hard.

Each morning I would show up at the portal, or the entry to the mine, at 7:00 A.M. It would take an hour to traverse down the seven miles of dark underground mine shafts and tunnels to arrive at the face of where the latest work was going on. Fortunately, we were also paid for the hour coming and going each day, in addition to the six hours of labor.

It was a forbidding environment lit only by small, dim, overhead bulbs and the lanterns on our helmets; wet, dank, and cold. Fortunately, I was not claustrophobic.

The miners were a close-knit community, and I found out quite by accident that they had an initiation rite, not unlike the cruel rituals that some fraternities enjoy foisting on new recruits. With that piece of insider information and my speed, I was lucky to escape my intended fate that first day of work.

I still don't know what the history of the ritual was, other than to humiliate its recipient. When you arrived on your first day at the tunnel, on your trek to the face of the dig, a group of men and/or boys would pull your pants down and rub cold, thick axle grease between your legs and all over your genitals. However, with my speed, I was able to run like hell and escape their clutches.

I could easily imagine the awful feeling of working all day in long bib overalls while the black grease slowly worked its way around to my rectum, down my legs, and over my privates, squishing between my legs with every step.

My job was to either lay new track as the mine became deeper and deeper, or to haul the immense timbers into position to form the bracing structure that kept the mountain from falling down on top of us all. I did this for the first half of the summer and then got a reprieve to work outside shoveling sand.

Every week new mountains of sand would be delivered to the site adjacent to the mine. Next to these enormous piles were large heaters. Once again, I was shoveling, only this time it wasn't garbage, it was tons of sand. We would throw shovel after shovel onto the bed of the heaters where it would dry out enough so that it could be used on the wheels of the carts—the drier and grittier, the better.

Each cart had a small receptacle just above the wheels, which held a couple of cups of sand. This would trickle out onto the slick tracks to help slow down the carts.

The labor was difficult, but I enjoyed the upper body workout from lifting the heavy shovel all day, and the camaraderie of the other workers helped to overcome the boredom of the monotonous task.

One funny story that comes to mind when I remember those days working in the mine and living with my grandparents, was the time I found a basket full of whiskey bottles in the fruit cellar. When I had been living with my aunt and uncle in California, Grandmother used to send us fruitcakes every year. Now, these weren't your standard re-gifting fruitcakes, the kind you can drive a nail with. No, these were the best tasting cakes I'd ever eaten. Every time I dug into one, after sneaking three or four pieces, I would just feel so right with the world, even a little lightheaded with happiness.

It turned out it wasn't happiness that made me lightheaded; it was one of the ingredients in Grandma's cakes. After I'd been living with her and Grandpa for about three weeks, she sent me down into the cellar to get some bleach. As I was rooting around down there, I saw a large wicker basket crammed with half-full whiskey bottles, and I thought, *What in the world?* When I returned upstairs, I asked Grandma why there was a basket of whiskey bottles in the basement, and why none of them was empty. She replied, "Oh, those are your Grandpa's. He's not supposed to drink, so he sneaks it a little here

and there and then he hides the bottles. I always find
them when he's finished about half of one, and I add it to
my collection down in the cellar."

"What are you saving them for Grandma?" I asked.

"I use them in my fruitcakes. I put a lot of it into the
mix; helps to preserve them nicely."

The point to all this background information is that,
from the earliest time I can remember, I always adapted
well to my circumstances, no matter what they were.

I used the skills God gave me to my advantage and
because I was surrounded by positive people, I felt that I
could do anything I put my mind to. I knew I would
never be fearful just because I happened to find myself in
a strange or difficult situation or place.

I remember my first year at BYU. Though I had come
from a family of Mormons (remember Great-grandmother Soffe who walked all the way to Utah?), I had
seldom attended the Church until I got to BYU. Every
student, regardless of his or her major, is required to take a
religion class each year. It was in those classes that I began
to develop my faith, and it was at that time that I finally
started asking myself some serious questions about who I
was and what I wanted to do with my life. The answers
didn't come to me overnight, but they did arrive.

For three years at BYU, I was a physical education
major. My wish was to become a coach and mentor, to
sort of repay what so many coaches had given me.

However, in the final analysis, I have to admit, the lure of money became more powerful and I ultimately changed my major to obtain a degree as a Chartered Life Underwriter (CLU), which sounds so dull now.

Life as an insurance executive

My first wife, El-Marie, and I were married in July of 1950 and what a lovely woman she was. I left BYU that same year during the Korean War. I was activated into the Air National Guard in 1951, where I learned to fly and where I got my first sales experience. In the evenings when our training was completed, I sold insurance in the barracks to the airmen. It wasn't long after I joined that our first daughter Melody was born.

Twenty months, six days, and three hours later, I was discharged.

After my stint in the service, I went back into the insurance business with New York Life. That year our second child, Billy, was born but only lived to be eleven months old. He died of a heart virus (crib death).

Later, my father-in-law, who was with Metropolitan Life in Blackfoot, Idaho, convinced me to join that firm and put my always-competitive nature to work learning the intricacies of agency management.

Not long after I joined Met Life, I became the president of the Life Underwriters Association.

Following that affiliation, I moved on to New England Life, the oldest chartered company in the country, and opened an office for them in Ogden, Utah. After that, I was recruited to become the Vice President and Director of Agencies for a small company called Western Empire Life.

In this new role, I was able to own shares in the company. My success and unusually high income allowed me to build a nice nest egg that I used to buy shares, which, in turn, appreciated quite nicely in just a short period of time.

By 1964, I was nearing my thirty-fifth birthday and now had more than fourteen years of experience in the industry and, in particular, with the three largest life insurance companies in America.

During that tenure, I had discovered two important things about insurance. First, I learned that by cutting operating costs, a small insurance company could compete with larger firms. Second, after buying mutual funds for years, I observed that life insurance and investment programs like mutual funds were essentially competing for the same dollars, which I determined was to the detriment of both the investors and the policyholders. *Why not combine both into one policy?* My motto would be, "Freedom through financial independence."

The idea of mating mutual funds and insurance wasn't a new idea, but my version would be. With a growing belief that financial security and personal freedom are inextricably intertwined and that security could best be achieved through a mutual funds/insurance program, contrary to what my employer believed (I knew he wouldn't go along with the idea), I decided to form my own company or find one that I could buy.

In the weeks that followed, I poured through the Life Insurance Corporation Register in the hopes of finding such a firm. For various reasons, most of the companies were rejected, until one day I came across one—Life Insurance Corporation of America, owned by Bankers Life and Casualty, which was owned by the fifth wealthiest man in America, John D. MacArthur. He eventually agreed to sell the company to me and my partners.

The sale price was $600,000. Investors would be needed to raise the capital. As we were about to go public, one of my partners wanted to bring another company into the fold, but I didn't trust the CEO, a rigid and unyielding sort of man. Eventually, I raised $1 million for the company and operated it for three years, along with my partners, but we began to fight over the involvement of the issue of adding another company. It looked as if it would be the deal breaker. And it was. I did not trust the man who was running the company and with my two partners voting against me in the majority, I decided to leave. Later the company was sold to a savings and loan.

The Mormon Church

During this time, because of my success, I was able to be very generous in my tithing to the Church to which I'd become devoted.

While in Church one day in 1965, I met Sister Clawson who was known as the angel of Temple Square, the area on which the Mormon Tabernacle is situated. She became a friend and mentor and with her help, I soon found myself serving as a tour guide, a highly desirable and fun position.

Because Sister Clawson had taken me "under her wing," she always made sure that when the most interesting people came to Temple Square, I would get my turn to meet them, and provide them with tours and some of the rich history of the Church.

One of those influential visitors was Minister Raghaven, who was the Minister of Public Safety and Foreign Affairs for India's Indira Ghandi. He had just come from meetings in Washington, D.C., and because he was fascinated with the Church, he asked many questions. When I asked him about his allure to the Church, Raghaven said, "Bill, did you know that the Mormon Church is noted for being one of the best organized societies for caring for their people in the world? People everywhere are impressed with their welfare programs and structures."

This important man was extremely impressed and I was proud of what he had to say about my Church.

After serving as a tour guide for approximately two years, in 1967 Emily Smith Stewart, the eldest daughter of George Albert Smith, former president of the Church, told me I was going to be called upon to be a Bishop of my local ward, in which resided many powerful and important people. Emily had had a revelation. And, not long thereafter, I was chosen, just as she'd told me.

Perhaps a little history is in order here. In the early 1890s, Utah was still not a state and, of course, the most powerful force, political or otherwise, in the territory was the Mormon Church.

In 1850, Brigham Young was the Territorial Governor, and it wasn't until the following year that the long-held practice of what was called Celestial Plural Marriages was ever made public. It had been practiced since the Church's inception and turned out to be a very unpopular practice outside of Utah. In fact, in 1856 the new Republican Party selected for its national platform a call to abolish the "relics" of barbarism, slavery, and polygamy.

In that same year, the second proposal for statehood was rejected due to growing anti-Mormon sentiments amid complaints that unbelievers were said to be mistreated and that the Territorial Government was a mere puppet for the real power or theocratic dictatorship directed by the leaders of the Mormon Church.

After a forty-seven-year struggle for statehood and seven attempts, President Cleveland issued a statehood proclamation, but only after the Mormon Church "publicly" disavowed the practice of polygamy, or plural marriages. However, in private the practice thrived and even drove many people "underground." In fact, John Taylor remained as President of the Church and had eight wives. To the public, however, it appeared he only had one.

I had always followed the doctrine of the Church to the letter of the "law," and I was aware that there were those who were practicing pluralism, but the subject was never actually raised in Church. The hierarchy had abandoned the practice in order to placate the rest of the country and to gain statehood. The practice had been forced out of public scrutiny, nevertheless, there were many priesthood (fundamentalist) groups in existence, comprised of those who had left the Church over this issue and others.

After I had been a Bishop for about a year, I was approached by my High Priest Quorum Teacher who told me, "Bishop, they have changed so many things in the Church in order that we may get along with the world, it would make Joseph Smith (founder) turn over in his grave."

At that point, I felt compelled to defend the Church, and to investigate the doctrine known as the "Fullness of the Gospel."

In the past, my friend, Emily Smith Stewart, had become the First Lady of the Church, following her mother's death in the '40s.

She was seventy-two at the time, and in ill health with no one to take care of her. I invited her to live in my home temporarily during which time we discussed the political maneuvering within the hierarchy of the Church.

The more I thought about the fighting and the changes, the more disillusioned I became, so much so that I decided to leave the Church. Shortly thereafter, I was excommunicated, having been told that if I didn't follow the "new" ways, I would never go to Heaven.

Leaving the Church

Leaving the Church pained me deeply. I gave it a great deal of credit for the values it instilled in my family and me. In fact, my wife, El Marie, and my three children continued to be involved with the Church.

It was 1969 and El Marie and I had been married for nineteen years. We had three children: Melody, Bonnie, and Kathy. That year we were divorced. When we parted, I gave her the house, a cabin, and a mountain lot we owned. I never worried about my ability to earn a living. In fact, I was immediately hired as the president of another insurance company in Utah.

In 1970, I retired from the insurance industry. It isn't surprising that during this time, I turned once again to my faith and sought to find groups of like-minded people. There were plenty of people who had gone "underground" when the Church capitulated to become a state, and that exodus continued into the early '70s.

> DON'T PUT YOUR LIMITS ON MY GOD. DON'T TELL ME WHAT I MUST BELIEVE. IF GOD'S GOING TO DO HIS WORK, HE MUST BE FREE. DON'T PUT HIM IN A LITTLE BOX. AND SAY YOU MUST BE ORTHODOX. FOR THE LOVE OF GOD'S UNLIMITED TO ME.
> (FROM THE SONG, "DON'T PUT YOUR LIMITS ON MY GOD.")
> —REVEREND PATRICIA CAMPBELL

After I left the Church, I began to associate with people who had left on similar grounds. That's when I met Dr. Rulon Allred who was head of a major priesthood group. Dr. Allred was probably the most spiritual man I had ever met; a kind, loving, and gentle soul as well as a physician and a born leader.

Unfortunately, there were also other groups filled with excommunicated members competing against Allred's group for leadership. Once again, I experienced the insidious politics of religion. One afternoon after I had attended a meeting with Dr. Allred, he was shot and murdered not fifteen minutes after I left. One of the men from a rival group was eventually arrested.

After that incident, I met a man named John Bryant who was the president of the Patriarchal Church of Christ. Bryant was the first person I had ever met who wrote through the spirit. In other words, he could call upon God, and conduct a dialogue, and then he would write those words.

Some of the members of these fundamentalist groups had multiple wives. The original intent of pluralism under the founder, Brigham Young, was for the men to provide teaching, a sense of community, and spiritual help to their wives, who might otherwise have remained single without much support.

The Church became that community of assistance and encouragement. In the traditional sense, the women choose which man's family she wants to join. In Mormon terms, this is called "sealing" them to the men. They are not technically or legally married and often don't even cohabitate with their "husbands" all the time.

That was the way of the original Church. When the female population far outnumbered the males, women were sealed to the men so that, in addition to being

Church law (a commandment from the book, Doctrine & Covenants), there was a practical side to pluralism.

Today, unfortunately, the politics and motivations of people in many of these fundamentalist groups often have different agendas and are receiving negative media coverage, and rightly so, for their ways are not what Brigham Young had envisioned.

It was at this time, while I was a member of the fundamentalist priesthood group, that I met Reta, a lovely and very bright woman that I married. She had been the top agent in my former insurance company. She had five children. In the next several years, Reta and I had a set of twin girls and two boys, raising the head count to nine.

We were not married in the traditional legal sense until later, but were joined by the priesthood. She had moved from Las Vegas and had purchased a small home with two bedrooms and an extra room in the basement in which to house our nine children and Reta's sister when she visited. It was cramped, but we were happy.

It was in this group that I met the four women who would be sealed to me over the years: Margaret, Lola, Lucille and Havah. I believed in the spirit of these unions and hoped I would be able to provide emotional and spiritual support to all of them.

Reinventing myself

Through an odd series of events, the next year Reta and I became involved in a new business, a unique idea at the time called timeshares, which involved selling shares of various condominiums and hotel rooms to investors. Each shareholder paid a set amount to own a block of time each year in either a condominium or hotel, generally in a resort or vacation locale.

The business began to look extremely bright when I met a contractor in Majorca, Spain, who was building resort condominiums. We struck a deal with the developer and, with a lot of planning, formed what was believed to be the first timeshare company. However, soon after our start-up, the Securities and Exchange Commission (S.E.C.) ruled that the investment concept was a security, which meant it had to be registered as a stock. We could not afford the attorneys and the fees and eventually Resorts International, now a billion-dollar company, stepped in and developed the concept. Today they have timeshares as well as many other resort properties worldwide.

It was time for us to move on to yet another new business. I had heard that land was selling for bargain prices in Park City, Utah, and so our new dream was to purchase land for a new home and buy and resell lots.

At that time, in the early '70s, in that area of the country, "do-it-yourself" home building was the craze. People would buy a lot and then go to any number of do-it-yourself builders to help them construct their homes. Usually, the company would do the foundation and framing work, leaving the owner to either finish the rest on his own, or hire the company to help with the more technical aspects such as electrical wiring and plumbing.

One such company, Capp Homes of Minneapolis, the largest and most successful company of its kind (do-it-yourself home building), helped us build our home. By the time we were nearly finished, I'd gained just enough knowledge of construction techniques that I felt qualified to take a job with Capp selling the building lots and new construction.

In 1979, after seven years of building over 400 homes, I met Webb Lowe, a former executive vice president with the MacDonald's food chain, who helped me to franchise the home-building business and take it national.

Within a year, I had embarked on my next career, that of homebuilder. Webb and I became friends and formed a company called Independent Homebuilders of America. Within the first two years, we had forty offices in ten Western states.

This venture was quite successful until the early 1980s when interest rates skyrocketed to 23 percent, effectively putting a firm damper on the entire building industry.

During the '70s, I was also very active with the priesthood group doing what I call missionary work, in a manner of speaking. I had my pilot's license and a plane, a Mooney single engine. For the previous five years, I had been flying some of the priesthood members down to a small town in Mexico called, Ozumba near Mexico City; where there was a colony of people like ourselves who had been cut off from the Church. Our goal was to support them spiritually as well as with business advice.

I'll never forget one trip. We were late getting started. By the time we were halfway down to Mexico City, the sun was setting. Then, in that area of Mexico, it was illegal to fly a single engine plane after dark.

One of our passengers was also a flight instructor. He wanted to pilot, so I climbed into one of the backseats. I only had what they call a visual flight rating anyway, meaning I wasn't supposed to fly on instruments. However, it got so black out, the instructor said he wasn't comfortable landing in the dark so we switched places. As soon as I climbed into the seat, I called the airport at San Luis Potosi on the radio. It looked like everything was going to be fine until the controller at the airport radioed back that they didn't have any lights. I don't even think the moon was visible that evening.

The six of us put our thinking caps on and came up with a solution. I radioed the controller back and asked him if they had any vehicles available. He said, yes they had several trucks, a couple of motorcycles and several cars, and then asked why.

I radioed him back, "Great. Why don't you line them up on both sides of the runway and turn on their headlights?"

We managed to land safely, but that wasn't the end of the story. Because we were flying in the dark, technically illegal, we were not only greeted by the headlights, but by a contingent of the army that wanted to search the plane for contraband—they thought we were drug smugglers. Silly me, I thought that people only smuggled drugs *out* of Mexico.

Within the hour, we were all lined up in front of the local magistrate and wound up paying a fine, which was actually a bribe, to be able to leave the next morning.

On yet another trip to the colony, we had a much bigger scare. When I started the engine that morning to let it warm up, it began making a funny sound like a faint "clank." I raced the engine a little to see if it was running properly. After a second the noise stopped, so I didn't give it any further thought.

There were four of us on that trip and as we lifted off the end of the runway at Mazatlan, and began to gain altitude, I heard the noise again, only this time it was louder and more consistent. That's when we began to lose speed. When we reached 2,500 feet, the plane stopped ascending and began to lose altitude rapidly; I was concerned that we might stall.

I knew that the Mooney had the longest glide path ratio of any small plane, which meant it would sail fairly well, even if we lost power. The one thing I was apprehensive about was our inevitable landing. Most of the area around us was comprised of ancient volcanic rock, not exactly an ideal material on which to land.

Fortunately, I managed to barely nurse the plane back to the airport, and all the while, the three brothers in the backseat were calmly discussing what we would do when we got to the colony.

Brother Allred later told me that he wasn't concerned because he knew it wasn't his time. I brought up this story to illustrate just how spiritual these men were. Brother Allred wasn't afraid of dying. He always just let go and let God handle things. He trusted in God with a strength I had never experienced. He was absolutely fearless because of his faith.

In 1982, Reta and I divorced. Among our other disagreements, she wanted to remain in the Mormon Church, which I, and of course, had already moved beyond years before.

Reta took all the children who weren't in college, and I let her take over my contractor's license. Considering the state of the industry, I didn't want to have anything more to do with home building at that point.

She and the children moved to St. George, Utah, and all of them ended up living in beautiful large homes which Reta and the children built. I moved to Las Vegas that year to be closer to them.

Although Reta was a bright person and became very successful at developing properties, she could be very authoritarian.

On one occasion, an employee in the construction company, who was also a priest (but a little rough around the edges because he liked to drink and smoke), was arrested and called me to bail him out.

I couldn't get back from the city, so I asked Reta if she would go. She did, taking our two boys with her. When they arrived at the small jail, she allowed the boys to accompany her to the cell where our young employee was being held.

"You see that," she said. "If either of you ever ends up in here, I'll leave you here."

Reta was, and is, the most dedicated mother and grandmother I've ever known, and I am most grateful for all she did for our family. I was always in awe of her ability to handle so many children and tasks simultaneously. It certainly rubbed off, because all of our children are quite successful and highly respected in their professions, the family, and Church.

From 1983 to 1993, I lived a life of semi-retirement just ninety-five miles south of where my children were living. (Reta now has eighteen grandchildren; I have nineteen, plus two great-grandchildren).

Chapter Three

The Invention of Alcalert

In 1989, I reinvented myself once again. This time, my new venture would prove to be the forerunner to the protocol that would eventually save my life—what we now call the Parkimin Sprays.

While living in Las Vegas, I got to know a number of the highway patrol officers and casual conversations often ended up on the same subject; drunk driving and the high mortality rates in Nevada. It seemed odd to me that with all the technological advances that were coming on line in the late '80s, something couldn't be invented to solve at least part of the problem.

Then, one afternoon, while at an office Christmas party, I had a glass of champagne, but I was certainly not intoxicated. Almost immediately afterwards I was driving home when I ran what I thought was a yellow light. Sure enough, not a block later, the bright red, yellow, and blue lights of a squad car appeared in my rearview mirror.

After I pulled over and handed my license to the officer, he asked me to step out of the car. I was a little chagrined because the police don't generally ask you to get out of your vehicle unless they suspect you of driving under the influence of something.

Upon exiting the vehicle, he asked me if I'd been drinking. He added, "You smell of alcohol," and indeed it had only been a few minutes since I'd imbibed the glass of champagne at a Christmas office party.

As my feet hit the pavement, my right foot came out from under me and I slipped and fell (I had on a brand new pair of leather-soled cowboy boots). Of course, he immediately assumed I was drunk.

As I began to stand up he said, "Okay fella, just stand there by your car. I'm going to have to test you." At that point, he pulled a small breathalyzer machine out of his car and administered the test, which consisted of my blowing into a short tube. Fortunately, since I'd only had the one glass of champagne, I was exonerated.

This experience solidified my resolve to find something that could alert a person if he or she was intoxicated. It occurred to me that if people who had been drinking could test themselves for blood alcohol levels prior to getting into a car, they might not drive. If only half the potential "drunk" drivers opted not to go out onto the roads, I would be doing mankind a great service and making good money in the bargain. In addition, with my connections, I felt I could easily obtain endorsements from the Highway Patrol and other law enforcement agencies in order to sell coin-operated breathalyzers.

I bought fifteen of the machines, and put them into high-end taverns. My intentions were to pay a commission to the waitresses for every bottle of spray that they sold as a result of the tests that indicated their patrons were intoxicated. They kept track of their sales by removing a tiny red bonus sticker we'd placed on each bottle, then they would turn those in for their commissions.

Unfortunately, due diligence, research, and early tests showed that most people who determined they were over the legal limit with such a device, still got into their cars and drove. In fact, the more inebriated they became, the more likely it was that they would ignore the evidence altogether.

So, I decided to turn lemons into lemonade. I reasoned that if people would not stop driving, even when they knew they were drunk, perhaps I ought to invent something that would sober them up quickly. I met with a pharmacologist who was involved in nutrition. He gave me a quick course on how the body processes alcohol, what it destroys in the system, and how the body uses it.

Without going into a great deal of scientific background, he told me I needed heavy doses of vitamins, particularly B vitamins and B-12 that act on the central nervous system. It was equally essential to incorporate vitamins A and E into the mix.

We also discovered that the Breathalyzer machines measure levels of "flammability" in the mouth and throat, which is why, even after a single drink, a person could be perceived by the machine to be intoxicated.

My first efforts involved combining the appropriate ingredients in a tablet or pill form, but that proved ineffective. Research showed that less than 10 percent of the necessary vitamins ever found their way into the bloodstream because most of the nutrients were not being absorbed in the stomach, liver, and intestines but eventually ended up in the sewer system (they pass through the body almost entirely).

In order for the vitamins to do their job sobering people up, they would have to enter the bloodstream rapidly and in full strength. That left only two solutions; an injectable delivery was immediately dismissed, of course, but the second option would prove to be revolutionary and quite effective. That is when my friend Webb introduced me to a company that made vitamin sprays.

After some experimentation with different ingredients with this company, we came up with a spray to sober people up. I named it Alcalert. It came in the form of a small atomizer from which a person could easily and quickly deliver the ingredients with a few pumps on the tongue or "alpha-lingualy" where it would bypass the stomach and intestines and go directly into the bloodstream within two minutes.

From my discussions with the pharmacologist, I knew that the vitamin A and E oils, being fat soluble, insulated the alcohol from the brain, attaching themselves to the alcohol molecules and specific receptors in the brain. Since the vitamins are not flammable and the receptors are isolated, scientifically speaking, the person could sober up rapidly.

The first guinea pigs for the invention were my colleagues, Webb Lowe and Joe Dehl. I still had leftover breathalyzer equipment and decided to test it on them.

At noon the next day they both began drinking and continued to do so through the afternoon. Joe used the spray a little at a time as he drank. Webb didn't use it at all until he'd consumed about five glasses of wine.

After an hour and a half, I tested both men. Joe never did get drunk, but Webb blew a .25 percent, nearly two and a half times the legal limit in most states.

When Webb finally used the spray and we retested him within a few minutes, his Breathalyzer test showed his level had dropped to an astounding .03 percent.

In addition, I gave some of the sprays to one of my highway patrol friends, and he reported using it on several of his inmates who had been brought in on DUIs. He told me that they appeared to sober up completely within minutes of using the spray. We were most definitely on to something. The year was 1989.

Chapter Four

All my dreams are waiting for me to come true

Suddenly I was in a new business altogether. With the help of my daughter, Melody, and my friends, Don Dowell and Leigh Carrol. I was once again making lemonade, real sweet lemonade, in the form of vitamin sprays.

The lemons, or the failure of the Alcalert project, only increased my creative energy. Webb's blood alcohol level dropped from .25 percent to .03 percent, an astounding decrease in just minutes. His level registered only .03 percent, but that wasn't the real blood alcohol level because the vitamins and amino acids in the spray were only masking the true levels and also covering up the breath odor. He was essentially cheating the machine.

I LOVE ME ENOUGH . . . TO REMEMBER THAT THE MOST LOVING THING I CAN DO FOR OTHERS IS TO BECOME THE BEAUTIFUL PERSON I AM MEANT TO BE. LOVING ME ALLOWS ME TO LOVE YOU AND ALL OF LIFE. I BECOME A GIFT TO THE UNIVERSE.

Further research showed that the liver still had to process the alcohol out, which takes hours. Essentially, ingested alcohol goes to the cerebellum in the brain, which sets off electric impulses, which in turn affects your motor skills.

The Alcalert also goes to the cerebellum, along with its B complex and A & E oils, and insulates and nourishes the brain. This diminishes the effects on motor skills. Essentially, it does bring you back to neutral faster than if you hadn't taken it but, technically, the person still has some level of alcohol in the bloodstream; it just doesn't register on the Breathalyzer. The "real" level would still show up in a urinalysis or blood test, but his motor skills were much improved.

Another thing we discovered was that since the B-12 molecule is so large, the first attempts to use the sprays "sublingually" (*under* the tongue) did not work as well as spraying it on *top* of the tongue. The reason for this was simple and had been overlooked by some of the other companies that were selling various sprays.

When the spray is applied *under* the tongue, where the saliva glands are most active, most of it is actually diluted. The results are much different than taking a pill—where most of the substance passes through the body without being absorbed.

When the spray is applied to the *top* of the tongue and then massaged by the tongue into the cheeks where those larger capillaries are most prevalent, the ingredients go directly into the bloodstream.

Our first thoughts were that we could market it as a deterrent to a DUI (Driving Under the Influence). Of course, there were two problems with that. First, it was wrong to help drunks avoid arrest, and there was also the liability issue. If someone thought that Alcalert would speed up his or her recovery, when it didn't work as fast as they thought it should, everyone involved would either be ripe for a lawsuit or our insurance rates would skyrocket.

The lemonade came when the patrolmen told me that regardless of how well or poorly it worked for those who were inebriated, the spray made them feel better, more alert, with more energy; it seemed to give them a boost on those long shifts. That gave me an idea. We had already invested a great deal of money in research and development of the sprays. Since I still had 50,000 units in storage, why not just change the name and market it as an energy spray (which is what it was).

Our first marketing efforts involved producing an infomercial. We hired an agent to write and film a two-minute spot, which was then sent into a production company to edit and place with the appropriate media. Unfortunately, the production company went bankrupt before we could have the spot aired. We had poured a great deal of money into the effort and now had to think of something else.

At the time, my daughter Melody had been in market-ing with Shaklee, an enormous multi-level marketing company, and we came up with the name of Revitalizer and a plan to sell it through a multi-level marketing process.

In a multi-level marketing plan, each salesperson not only sells the product to a buyer, he or she signs up buyers as new sales agents, who in turn operate under them.

Each salesperson is paid a commission on his or her own sales, as well as on the sales of all those representatives below him or her. This became our marketing vehicle to promote Revitalizer.

New sales reps were buying the products and signing up even more sales forces in droves. From the outset, we were doing quite well. The company was named Trendsetters.

In 1995, Melody and I split from Don and formed our own company, MJB Global, Inc., and we moved to more efficient facilities in Southern California. Shortly thereafter, I began to develop other sprays, all various combinations of natural vitamins and amino acids, each for different applications.

By early 1997, the company was doing extremely well with a full line of successful products. I was on top of the world until one night, as I began to address the audience at my high school reunion, I experienced the violent tremor in my right hand, the first symptom of Parkinson's.

Chapter Five

I have what?

As mentioned earlier, I was initially diagnosed with "essential tremors," not much to worry about However, months later, and after further tests, it was confirmed that I had Parkinson's.

The prognosis was bleak and I became progressively worse, to the point that I could barely roll over in bed. By 2000, I began to be very concerned and had little hope, something I now consider the most vital aspect of the healing process. Not one of my doctors expressed any hope, which I now see was a precipitating factor in the worsening of my condition.

As you will see in Chapter Six, there is a biology or a physical reality to the phenomenon of hope that can lead to complete remissions and cures for just about every illness known to man.

Hope begins with an absolute belief that you *will* get better, which leads to an expectation and then an unyielding desire. None of these things can take place when you are told by a person you can trust (doctor, physician, friend, or other "authority") that you will not get better.

Eventually, I gave up the day-to-day operation of the company and began to spend more and more time at my home office. Then I began to give up on myself. At some point I realized I was wallowing in self-pity, and that irritated me to no end!

It was then that I began my research odyssey. Specifically, I became a voracious reader. First, there were the hundreds of existing books on the current "realities" of mainstream thinking on the subject of Parkinson's, most touting the identical hopeless medical establishment mantras: learn to live with it, treat it with pills, make yourself as comfortable as possible, and get ready to die.

An amino acid compound in pill form, known as Sinamet, is the "gold standard" today for the treatment of Parkinson's and so I began taking that as I initially believed there was little else I could do. Treating the disease with Sinamet has its pluses and minuses. On the positive side, it does help to alleviate symptoms. It can decrease tremors and help increase appetite and range of motion. However, once again, with a pill, since it is ingested through the stomach and the intestines, little of the compound reaches the blood stream and, hence, the brain. In addition, the effects generally come in what I refer to as "highs," or all at once. These good effects diminish quickly, leaving the patient in the grips of the symptoms once again. Timing *when* to take the pill and just how long the effects will last depends upon several factors, all quite unpredictable.

Another treatment that is currently being used was developed by a world-renowned neurologist by the name of Dr. Perlmutter whose protocol consists of injections of an amino acid called glutathione. As mentioned in the publisher's letter at the beginning of this book, the injections have a powerful and immediately positive effect. Patients go from being nearly incapacitated to an almost normal range of motion within minutes of receiving the injections.

However, this high is only temporary and within twenty-four to forty-eight hours, the sufferer is nearly immobile again. Shots must be repeated three to five times a week at a cost of approximately $100 per injection. The obvious reason the glutathione works is because it is injected and goes into the bloodstream and then almost immediately to the brain.

The "blood brain barrier" surrounds the central nervous system and will allow only certain things into the brain from the blood. Neurotransmitters do not cross the blood/brain barrier into the brain. This means if you give neurotransmitters to patients orally or by IV, they either don't get enough of the product, or the result, as in Dr. Perlmutter's patients, is that they get a large jolt or high that diminishes rapidly. Administering neurotransmitter levels is not an option for raising their levels in the brain. You must give the body the "nutrients" it needs to produce those neurotransmitters (vitamins, amino acids, and minerals). These nutrients do effectively cross the blood/brain barrier into the brain where they are then synthesized into neurotransmitter molecules.

From my experiments with Sinamet and my discovery of Dr. Perlmutter's work, it became obvious to me that whatever the treatment consisted of, **it had to be delivered into the bloodstream quickly, and it had to be done in a time-released manner to maintain a reliable and steady effect throughout the day. It also had to have the right combination of "nutrients" that would produce the desired neurotransmitters to the brain.**

Getting worse

As I grew worse, my life was becoming increasingly chaotic. I know the intellect resists chaos, but that resistance only works, or is acceptable, if we know about the chaos in advance and can prepare for it. Like taking a roller coaster ride that we *know* might be scary, as long as we realize it is under control and will end in a safe manner, we are prepared for the thrills—that is, our intellect can control our emotions. My deterioration over more than two years was not something for which I was prepared.

THE ONLY THING YOU CAN KEEP IS WHAT YOU GIVE AWAY.

However, I'd already been to the specialists, and they all felt it was hopeless. By this time, I had realized through personal experience, research, and reading that the predominant form of health-care in this country is *symptom* not *preventative* based. We treat the symptoms with drugs, radiation, or surgery once it's progressed far enough to become uncomfortable or unbearable. I was at the unbearable stage.

In general, our medical establishment treats illness and disease by employing drugs and treatments that are designed to produce opposite effects than those displayed by the symptoms. In other words, they might give you a sleeping pill to treat insomnia, or an alkaline for acid indigestion. In their minds, the worse your symptoms, the more you need drugs, invasive surgeries, or chemicals.

We are also taught that we human beings are the sum of our individual parts, which accounts for the massive "specialization" that is the center point of our medical establishment. Each of these "specialists" (be that a cardiologist; podiatrist; or eye, ear, nose, and throat specialist), has his or her own story or myth about patients' body parts. These individuals are keener on a particular organ or system than they are about how the body/mind functions as a whole.

I was beginning to understand that the status quo was not what I needed. I needed to use all my powers—spiritual, mental, emotional and physical to treat *myself*. I knew that these aspects of me were inseparable, and I knew I had to educate myself.

Once I'd gone through hundreds of books, I decided my only alternative was just that, *alternative* thinking. How could I use my spirit, mind, and body to defeat Parkinson's?

My research and the advice from a few of my friends led me directly to Dr. Wayne Dyer. I subsequently met Dr. Deepek Chopra, who had been the Chief of Staff at New England Memorial Hospital in Boston, but was now located just down the street from my home in La Costa, California. Chopra's book, *Ageless Body, Timeless Mind* affected me quite profoundly. I not only read his books, I traveled all over the country listening to him in seminars. He subsequently became good friends with Dyer.

These concepts led me in turn to Candace B. Pert, Ph.D., Donald M. Epstein, and even the T.V. celebrity, Montel Williams, who learned to manage multiple sclerosis with many of these techniques, about which I was learning.

Further readings included *Your Body Believes Every Word You Say*, by Barbara Hoberman Levine, and liter-

FORGIVENESS MEANS GIVING UP ALL HOPE FOR A BETTER PAST.

ally scores of other books, which I have listed in the resource section in the back of this book and on our Web site at **www.noparkinsons.net**.

With each book or tape, I became increasingly more hopeful. My new knowledge also took me along a physical path to a new exercise regimen and a new way of eating. All of what I was learning was not just through my mind; it was through my spirit, mind, and body. I was assimilating all of it as one cohesive entity.

However, I have to say that my own research, along with the help of chemists that my company, MJB, employed, would prove to be just as astounding as the concepts about body/mind and spirit that I was learning.

At some point, as I began to have more faith in my own powers (spiritually, mentally, and physically), I also began experimenting with a resource I had completely dismissed—my own company, MJB Global.

Chapter Six

**The answer to my research and prayers—
Parkimin Plus Neutraceutical Sprays**

I knew that Sinamet worked in a limited capacity, and I understood the value of glutathione when I realized that the key to delivering these and other compounds into the blood stream and the brain was through a time-released vehicle that could be sprayed directly into the mouth, we began experimenting at MJB Global, Inc. with hundreds of various natural elements. Most were vitamins or amino acids. One was an element that stimulates the human growth hormone, or HGH, and there were various minerals as well.

Before we developed the Parkimin Sprays, I had written a confidential research and development proposal for MJB Global and Parkimin Technologies. This paper was written in 2002, and gives a brief explanation of the disease and the then current realities in terms of treatments:

> *Progress in the area of neurological diseases was not impressive until the late 1960s, when researchers identified a fundamental brain defect*

in all Parkinson's patients. This was the marked loss of brain cells that produce "Dopamine". The most affected area of the brain was apparently the "Substantia nigra" or the small pigmented area that connects the lower area of the brain to the upper area.

According to the National Institute of Neurological Disorders and Stroke (NINDS), Dopamine and other identified neurotransmitters are no longer produced by these cells and thus the smooth movement of muscles becomes greatly impaired. Scientists devoted the next few years to developing methods to re-introduce Dopamine and other identified neurotransmitter chemicals into the brain cells.

In the late 1970s, scientists determined that introduction of a related compound, "Levodopa or L-Dopa" into the fine minute blood cells of the brain would allow the brain to convert it to Dopamine. This natural substance of certain plants and animals was available for extraction, but was not so easily available for the brain to use.

By the late 1970s, several pharmaceutical houses were manufacturing L-Dopa product, which, according to the National Institute of Health (NIH), relieved Parkinson's symptoms such as shaking, slowness of movement, and stiffness. L-Dopa quickly became the "gold standard" for Parkinson's patients and others with neurological disorders. It remains so today in 2004.

However, the problems of absorption by the bloodstream into the brain are tremendous. According to studies, the L-Dopa is greatly absorbed through the gut and liver before it can reach the blood system of the brain. Indeed, according to NINDS, "Only 1 percent of the L-Dopa in each pill actually reaches the patent's brain." Thus, to show any positive effects, patients have to take large amounts of the drug, which in turn leads to all sorts of side effects, including nausea, sleeplessness and vomiting, as well as more tremors and even hallucinations.

Unfortunately, there are bad side effects to the oral administration of L-Dopa. Apparently, the longer it is taken, the more ineffective it becomes, and also the more it attacks critical enzymes for conversion to Dopamine.

The late '80s, and '90s saw research into other means of stimulating the brain cells to start producing Dopamine again. Since then, in addition to surgical implants of healthy nerve cells, special focus has been done on the brain cell mitochondria and their utilization of other proteins and amino acids, as well as enhancing direct delivery of the L-Dopa to the brain cells. Most recently, researchers are working with a "time released L-Dopa patch" which is being worn at the base of the brain.

Dr. Gary Null, in his **Ultimate Anti-Aging Program** (shown on a nationally featured PBS Documentary), discusses in detail several studies of Parkinson's patients and concludes that the problem is not the use of L-Dopa but rather, it is with the administration of effective amounts in sustainable balanced quantities. The American Parkinson's Disease Association (ADPA), in its well-circulated handbook on Parkinson's **Good Nutrition in Parkinson's Disease** discusses the problems associated with taking L-Dopa. The Association recommends everything from putting your tablets into a liquid form to spacing your intake of protein throughout the day so that "it doesn't interfere with L-Dopa absorption.

We (Bill Hansen and MJB Global) have concluded that the time has arrived for introducing our spray delivery system to patients with impaired neurological disorders. The introduction of this program begins with this book and will include our proprietary Parkimin Six Pack, a specially developed group of nutritional supplements, amino acids and enzymes, which assist the brain in maintaining good cell activity.

We have identified a group of twenty patients and are finalizing the serum uptake tests and protocol for the Phase I efficacy studies. While these studies are underway, we also plan on bench-scale development of Fava Bean Extractions, which are reportedly very high in Levodpa. It is our intention to deliver this "natural" form of L-Dopa in a spray that bypasses the stomach and liver and goes straight into the blood vessels in the brain. Thus, many of the problems cited above with conventional L-Dopa therapy could be alleviated and avoided.

Further, the following was an online article on the subject of drug dosages:

Future Tech: A Pill with Your Name On It. Microchips and micro muscles could spell the end of one-size fits-all medicine.
By Trevor Theime

When Robert Langer looks out the window of his lab on the edge of the Massachusetts Institute of Technology campus, he sees the future of medicine . . . .

Langer's team is one of several research groups nationwide developing programmable implants that could revolutionize the way drugs are administered and overcome one of the most common obstacles to effective medical treatment.

All too often, getting the right doses of a pharmaceutical to the precise target proves difficult. Pills are problematic because the digestive system breaks down many therapeutic compounds before they can reach the bloodstream. Injections bypass

*the stomach but are expensive and inconvenient, as
well as difficult to self-administer.*

*Worst of all, both needles and pills can cause
dangerous fluctuations of drug concentrations.
For example, too much insulin kills a diabetic; too
little can cause a coma.*

Getting much better

By mid-1999, I had managed to incorporate more than
100 ingredients into ten different sprays that I used reli-
giously about five times a day. Coupled with my spiritual
beliefs, my daily workouts, and a new diet, I began to
improve. By mid-2002, I had improved greatly, though I
would still experience tremors, especially if I was nervous. At the time of this writing, I still utilize the Sinamet
in small doses throughout the day in conjunction with
the sprays.

One day I had a real scare. Everything seemed to be
going quite well. I was in the shower and was about to
turn off the water when suddenly I couldn't move. It
really took me by surprise. I literally could not even turn
off the water! I told myself to relax, not to panic, and take
some slow deep breaths; very slowly, my muscles relaxed
slightly, just enough so that I could open the shower door
but I still couldn't walk, so I crawled ever so slowly to
where my bathrobe was lying across the toilet. I rolled
over on my side and managed to put my arms into the
sleeves. It must have taken me four or five minutes to

crawl the ten feet into the den where I managed to hold onto the phone and punch in my friend Donna's number, who came over immediately and helped me into bed.

Later that day, the problem subsided and I was completely mobile again. That kind of incident has never happened again, thank God. What it told me, however, was that my sprays still needed some work, which is when we began experimenting with the addition of more nutrients that we learned were needed to help the neurotransmitters cross the blood brain barrier into the brain.

> THE PAST IS HISTORY,
> THE FUTURE A MYSTERY.
> TODAY IS A GIFT.
> THAT'S WHY THEY CALL IT THE "PRESENT."

Once the sprays were working consistently, and while I was continuing with the Sinamet, I decided to visit a Dr. Gary Shima who was offering the same glutathione treatment that Dr. Perlmutter had been using. I wanted to see if injections of glutathione would enhance the results I was getting on my own.

After a couple of weeks of these injections, I was surprised to see they added nothing. I realized that the glutathione in the sprays, already being delivered in a day-long-time released manner, was doing the trick.

I must tell you, my story feels like living a miracle. For the most part, anyone who didn't know me would ever guess I have Parkinson's.

I live an eternally thankful and joyous life, now filled with hope—not just for me, but for thousands of others afflicted with this disease. I take every day as a gift to be savored, which is why I considered it my sacred contract to write this book and bring these discoveries out into the open.

I can now dance as I once did, particularly my favorite, the cha-cha, which challenges anyone who tries to master it, with very difficult, quick steps. I have regained all the weight I lost, I sleep so much better at night, and I work out three times a week in half-hour sessions.

I now call our MJB products Parkimin Sprays and we are currently developing new ones to treat Alzheimer's and many other neurological diseases such as ALS (Lou Gerhig's disease, Multiple Sclerosis) and others, all with similar approaches.

In a moment, in chapter seven, I will describe to you all that I have learned about the most important elements of my recovery—the Spirit, Mind and Body connection, and why and how it works, particularly in conjunction with the Parkimin Sprays.

Before we begin that chapter, let me say that though my protocol works very well for me and others (see the endorsements at the end of this book), research on the Parkimin Sprays still needs to be conducted, particularly clinical trials, which are quite expensive. It is true that since the sprays are all composed of natural elements, they need no FDA approval. However, in all honesty, we have not yet been able to be definitive as to which ingredients and portions are responsible for the amazing results I've enjoyed. Perhaps it is all of them or perhaps it is only a few; so I just continue to take them all.

Double-blind clinical tests are needed to determine just exactly what is working. In the meantime, I continue to experiment with adjustments to my protocol, using myself as the guinea pig. However, I can say one thing without hesitation; as effective as the Parkimin Sprays are, I know I would not have enjoyed such a rapid and full recovery without my faith in God and a full understanding and deployment of my Spirit, Mind and Body connection.

THE EVOLUTION OF A PERSON WITH PARKINSON'S . . . IN THE BEGINNING YOU ARE A PARKINSONIAN, AS YOU GET PROGRESSIVELY BETTER, YOU ARE A PARKIMINIMUM AND FINALLY, YOU ARE A PARKINONE

With that said, let's take a look at that connection.

Chapter Seven

The Spirit, Mind, Body Connection

As noted earlier my protocol includes not only the Parkimin Plus Sprays, but also a daily attentiveness to the Spirit, Mind, and Body connection.

I believe that through a knowledge and faith in this connection it is possible to "create" our own lives, to live exactly as we wish to live. I have a saying: *"All my dreams are waiting for me to come true."* In other words, I can become everything I can ever dream possible. In my case, of course, my passion is to be free of Parkinson's, and to once again, live a healthy and happy life.

> THE "WHAT" IS OUR JOB.
> THE "HOW" IS SPIRIT'S JOB.

My competitive nature, borne out of my many years of participation in sports, and, of course, the positive influences of so many beautiful people in my life, drove me to an answer.

When it appeared my dancing days were over, I was not happy. *Why did I bring this into my life?* I asked more times than I care to admit.

I remember praying to God on many occasions, asking only that He allow me the grace to regain my balance and to enjoy at least one bright spot in my life, dancing. Eventually, of course, my persistence and faith were rewarded.

How I got to this point is the subject of this chapter because I am convinced, beyond any doubt, that I would not be where I am (even *with* the use of the Parkimin Sprays), without learning to *"let go" and "let God,"* without making the connection between Spirit, Mind, and Body.

In its very simplest terms, this means a regimen of reflection, learning, inspiration, and knowledge (Mind); the proper nutrition and exercise (Body); and a deep awareness and faith (Spirit); knowing who I am and why I'm here.

Until these three elements of who you are come into harmony, you cannot be truly whole. One fuels the other in an endless loop. For the Mind to be clear and able to reflect and learn, the Body must be healthy and efficient. This means the proper diet coupled with a regular regimen of exercise. Nurturing your Spirit in daily devotions is essential as well.

> *I am independent of the good or bad opinions of others. I am beneath no one, nor above anyone. I am fearless in the face of any and all challenges.*
> From *SynchroDestiny* by Deepek Chopra

More than anything written on this subject (which is considerable), I would recommend you read the works of these authors: Dr. Deepek Chopra, Dr. Wayne Dyer, Candace B. Pert, Ph.D., and Carolyn Myss, Ph.D.

In order to get into this material, I will begin with the subjects of perception and behavior. Our perceptions about ourselves and the world around us are all *learned* behavior. These behaviors have been formed through conditioning by parents, teachers, friends, churches, and society.

Such conditioning has been going on (repetition) for thousands of years. In turn, *your* parents, teachers, and friends were conditioned by *their* parents, teachers and friends.

Unfortunately, many of the things we believe to be true are, in fact, false. Take, for instance, the notion that sickness and disease are inevitable, aging is inescapable, and stress is just a part of our hectic modern lives. We (all of us) have unwittingly agreed to participate in this fiction and it is time to discard these assumptions, along with many others, because the fact is, sickness, premature aging and stress are NOT inevitable. When we come to understand the Spirit, Mind, and Body connection and learn to let go, we will be able to live lives of exceptionally high physical and spiritual energy; we will be free from disease and stress; and we will discover the miracle of the possibilities of living in a world without arrogance, animosity, hate, greed or lust.

All of these negative emotions, what we call "stress," can be suppressed and virtually eliminated, for they are all illusions borne out of ego.

The Spirit, Mind, and Body Connection

*The **Body** is a remarkable vehicle, which allows us to feel physical sensations of pleasure and pain so we can learn from our experiences.*

*The **Mind** speaks to us with words, pictures, or images, which can translate into physical conditions in the body.*

*The **Spirit** is the life force within a body—the breath of life. We learn spiritual lessons related to love, compassion, and trust using Mind and Body. We are taught by feeling bodily experiences. **Mind** helps us to understand and create meaning, enabling us to grow as human (physical) and spiritual beings. **Spirit** is the part of us that observes, knows, grows and loves.*

—Barbara Hoberman Levine

Startling new discoveries

Perhaps one of the most critical research developments in the field of Mind/Body study was the discovery of neurotransmitters, particularly endorphins. Neurotransmitters are the chemical messengers that the brain uses to communicate with the body.

In 1986, Dr. Candace Pert published the first evidence suggesting that neurotransmitters, which also play an essential role in regulating the internal physiology of the body, had specific receptor sites throughout the body. According to Pert:

Neurotransmitters in the brain send and receive messages between cells that trigger the release of neurohormones, which then travel throughout the bloodstream to receptor sites in specific organs.

Research also shows that certain neurotransmitters, such as endorphins, play a role in mediating the stress response. Endorphins affect sensory states such as relief of pain and fatigue, and feelings of energy. They are found in high concentrations in the pituitary, the gland that is responsible for secreting the hormones that regulate bodily functions.

This information not only supported the concept of a Mind/Body connection, it also identified a mechanism for psychophysiological communication; in other words, the language the mind uses to communicate with the body!

Essentially the brain uses electrical impulses, while the organs of the body use chemical reactions to communicate.

According to Pert, research seems to strongly indicate the following:

- *The mind and body are intimately connected*
- *The mind and body communicate with one another via a complex mechanism of electrical and chemical messages*

- *The brain regulates the body via this electro-chemical mechanism*
- *The brain, the immune system, and the neuroen-docrine system are also interconnected via this mechanism*
- *The brain, via the hypothalamus and its produc-tion of neurohormones, plays a role in triggering and mediating the stress response*
- **It is possible to gain voluntary control over your immune system and your negative emotions**

In another portion of her book, Pert states:

> *Emotions are at the nexus between matter and mind, going back and forth between the two and influencing both. Thus, it could be said that the traditional separation of mental processes, includ-ing emotions, from the body is no longer valid.*

Dr. Pert's discoveries should not really surprise us. She and many other researchers have provided us with the evidence of what many people suspected for cen-turies: that the body is not a mindless machine; the body and mind are one. Her research simply validates what Eastern philosophers, shamans, and other alternative practitioners have been telling us for centuries; that our biochemical messengers act with intelligence by communicating information through a vast complex of conscious and unconscious activities at any one moment.

Again, in Dr. Pert's book, she says:

> *We can no longer think of emotions as having less validity than the physical, but instead must see them as cellular signals that are involved in the process of mind into matter.*

Essentially, it isn't mind *over* matter, it's mind *with* matter.

According to Dr. Chopra, in his introduction to Dr. Pert's book, *The Molecules of Emotion:*

> *This transfer of information takes place over a network linking all of our systems and organs, and engaging all of our molecules of emotion, as the means of communication. What we see is an image of a "mobile brain"—one that moves throughout our entire body, located in all places at once, not just in the head.*
>
> *This bodywide information network is ever-changing and dynamic, infinitely flexible. It is one gigantic loop, directing and admitting information simultaneously and intelligently guiding what we call life.*

Where and when did we all come to believe the myth that the Mind and Body are separate, or that every disease can be traced to a physical cause?

In his book, *Healing Myth, Healing Magic*, Donald Epstein writes:

> *The myth that every disease can be traced to a physical cause is part of a cultural hallucination that began years ago.*
>
> *In the seventeenth century, Rene Descartes, the French philosopher and mathematician, advanced the idea that anything objective, material, and measurable belonged to science; while the subjective, spiritual, and immeasurable belonged to the realm of religion and the Church. His ideas were further advanced by philosophers who taught that anything pertaining to the human mind should be relegated to the field of psychology.*
>
> *Philosophical concepts relating to the body, mind, and spirit were divided into separate 'camps' as proponents of each had their own view on the primacy of their story.*

More recently, scientists like Candace Pert and others, suggest that with every emotion we experience, certain tissues, including nerve cells and circulating white blood cells, vibrate at a particular frequency associated with a chemical (or peptide) attaching to the surface of the cell.

It could be said that the "tone" of the cell membrane, its biochemical interactions with neuropeptides, and its energy circulation and vibration *are* our emotions. Thus, the physical and emotional are both aspects of the same process. Likewise, what is called "spiritual" is at least partly an awareness of subtle energy in the body associated with certain peptides being activated in the brain.

To my own personal way of thinking, one of the most important statements from the list of findings on the previous page is this: **It is possible to gain voluntary control over your immune system and your negative emotions**. I am living proof. It is imperative however, that in order to do this, one must balance Spirit, Mind and Body. When you are in balance, your body will heal itself. In my case, the use of the Parkimin Sprays is part of that balance (body and diet).

It doesn't matter which religion you belong to. It is only important that you agree that we humans are aware creatures with free will, and that we are all one. In other words, we have the ultimate power to make choices every second, every day of our lives. It is possible, given the Spirit, Mind, and Body connection to take control over your immune system, indeed your entire life. Given the right choices, nothing is impossible. For example, consider this clinical study:

"Realization techniques help cancer patients."
London, April 15, 1999, Reuters.

Cancer patients can literally "think" themselves to a stronger immune system using relaxation and guided imagery techniques, a British researcher said on Saturday.

Professor Leslie Walker, the Director of the Institute of Rehabilitation and Oncology Health at the University of Hull in northern England, said that psychological techniques can also help patients better cope with disease.

Walker and his colleagues tested relaxation techniques on eighty women suffering from breast cancer. They presented their findings to the Annual Meeting of the British Psychological Society. All of the women received standard medical treatments for breast cancer, but half were randomly selected for training in muscular relaxation, guided imagery, and cue-controlled relaxation.

Guided imagery involves imagining the body's natural defenses battling the cancerous cells. In cue-controlled relaxation, patients learn to relax by thinking of special words. When the researchers tested all the women, they found that those practicing the relaxation techniques had a higher number of important immune system cells.

These results demonstrate that, even in patients with large tumors receiving immunosuppressive treatment (chemotherapy, surgery, radiotherapy), relaxation therapy and guided imagery can produce powerful immunological changes, Walker said.

The number of studies that document the Mind's ability to change how the Body works are literally countless. Think of the millions of people throughout the world who use various forms of meditation to slow down their heart rates, lower their blood pressure, and eliminate anxiety. These individuals turn these "learned" disorders into normal responses.

On a deeper level, we've all heard the stories of how cancer patients, who have a high expectation that they will recover statistically stand a far greater chance of recovering than those who live in doubt and despair about their futures.

GURU
GEE, YOU ARE YOU!
G.U.R.U.

WHAT THE MIND CAN CONCEIVE, THE BODY CAN ACHIEVE.

In addition, of course, there is further evidence of the Mind/Body connection known as the "placebo effect." A benign or fake drug is used in research to study the effects of real drugs on different sets of patients. One group is given a real drug, the other a placebo.

Repeatedly, these kinds of studies show that from 30 percent to 50 percent of the time, the patients in these studies who received a placebo (believing they were getting the real thing) experienced the same pain relief or rate of recovery as the group that received the real drug. And there are many documented cases of patients who have even experienced total remissions from advanced malignancies (cancers) by merely receiving injections of sterile saline solutions that they were told (and they "believed") were actually powerful anticancer drugs. Because they *believed* they would get better—*they did.*

Inversely, there are many cases of patients who have been incorrectly diagnosed with a life-threatening disease and told they had only a short time to live, only to die within that specific short timeframe; and for doctors to then discover they had absolutely no disease whatsoever. If you truly believe you're going to die, you probably will. If you believe you'll get better, in all likelihood, you will.

The biology of hope

Just as there is a neurochemical cause and effect associated with fear, there is a similar biology to hope. In the natural instinct of fear, or the fight or flight instinct, the brain sends messages along neural pathways, communicating with the various organs of our body. Cortisol and other powerful hormones and chemicals are immediately flushed into our bloodstream, preparing our muscles and other functions for fight or flight. This is an autonomic response. In other words, it happens automatically when you are fearful.

Like everything about us, there is a neurobiological reason for all of our thoughts and actions, including the emotion of hope, which is made up of two parts: *affective* or emotional; *cognitive* thought or logic.

Like the studies previously discussed, when people believe they will get better, more often than not, they do. Moreover, when they believe they are going to die, they often do. This occurs not just because they are emotionalized, but also because powerful physical transformations are occurring in their bodies. The formula goes something like this:

Hope = Absolute belief + expectation + desire.

When you hope for something, your mind begins to marshal information and data relevant to a desired future event. In the case of illness, that would be a cure.

The first thing that happens is your mind generates a different vision of your condition, a different vision than the one you originally had when you discovered you were ill. Generally this vision comes as a result of information you are given by a doctor or some other perceived "authority."

If you "absolutely" believe this source (let's say it's a physician renowned for curing your particular disease), then your mind begins to take comfort, your system is alerted and is energized and your mood begins to elevate. That is why we often refer to this feeling as being "lifted by **hope**," or as if on wings.

The two parts of your brain—cognitive and affective—now are working in harmony.

Hope is different from blind optimism: It brings reality into sharp focus. The chemical reactions in the body,
such as endorphins (the feel good hormone), which are
now flushed into the bloodstream temper panic and
despair and help to encourage the process of rational
deliberation so that you can think clearly. **Hope** helps us
to temper fear and to recognize dangers and then bypass
or endure them. This in turn just reinforces your belief.

While there is a "fear" center (the amygdala), in the
brain, there is no "hope" center; rather, the emotion of
hope is an intricate process wherein the brain communi-
cates with the body in an electrochemical fashion.

The key, and this is very important, is that you first
have to *believe* that you are going to get better.

For many who cannot see **hope**, their vision is blurred
because they *believe* they are unable to exert any level of
control over their circumstances. This is where the physician, healer, or other authority comes in.

Unfortunately, with all the wonderful things that
modern medicine has come up with, hope is not at the
forefront. You've already read the diagnosis I was given
when the doctors first discovered I had Parkinson's—
hopeless, treat it as best we can with drugs, prepare to
die—not exactly an uplifting prognosis.

Hope begins with the healer and the patient communicating. It takes more than mere words to communicate
the information that is needed to alter negative emotions
or despair. For a physician, healer, counselor, or minister
to set the chain of hopeful events into motion, he or she

must first have hope and believe in a positive outcome. He or she must not only communicate this in words, but also through his or her eyes and emotions.

In addition, of course, there are alternatives to what doctors say, and that is what this entire book is about—Spirit. Many of us turn to our faith for hope. We learn to *let go* and *let God*. We trust this power with our entire being.

Hope= Absolute belief in God, doctors, counselors, and other authorities, plus expectation coupled with desire.

It has also been proven that *fighters*, people who get "Hoppin" mad and decide to take matters into their own hands, tend to experience a greater rate of cure than those who give up and acquiesce to the doctor's recommended regimen. I was never prone to anger but my frustration with my limitations had the same effect. It drove me to all my research and learning.

> THE BRAIN IS AN ORGAN, THE MIND IS ITS ACTIVITY; THE PRESENT IS ITS PRODUCT.

But, of course, the paradox of "modern" medicine is that truly out-of-the-box thinking is rarely welcomed at first, no matter who proposes the ideas. Protecting the prevailing paradigm, science moves slowly because it doesn't want to make mistakes. We are not yet a society of preventative medicine. We just treat the symptoms, which only means you already have the disease.

No, it is far more important to begin with a belief in your own potential and the power of the Spirit to move you—

Mind and Body together in a cohesive and powerful healing machine—rather than wait for modern medicine to
climb aboard. **Begin with the medicine of hope.**

The power of the human mind never ceases to amaze
me. Current research in the Body/Mind interaction con-
firms that we are only as healthy and fulfilled as the quality
of our thoughts. **Our thoughts are a form of energy that
interact and change matter.** Negative thoughts tend to
have a negative effect on your immune system and your
mind. Positive thoughts tend to reap positive rewards. In
addition, negative thoughts held long enough, tend to
become words, which further exacerbates the situation. **We
speak both good and bad into existence.**

It is this simple: Where your interest lies, your mind
thrives. When your mind is absorbed and focused, it
doesn't wander or become so easily distracted or begin to
dwell on negatives. In my case my complete focus 24/7
was on healing myself.

Your Body Believes Every Word You Say, by Barbara
Hoberman Levine, is a phenomenal book that I consider
a must read for anyone seeking to get onto a permanent
positive track in life. In it, she asks:

> *Can you guide the inner intelligence that controls
> the automatic functions and behaviors of your body?
> Can you choose your level of health or illness? To the
> last question, the answer is YES, to a large degree.
> Dis-ease is a process over which you can have more
> control by carefully choosing your thoughts, your
> words, your attitude, and your actions.*

When you are responsible, you have the choice of altering the way that you think. Speak and act in order to change the effect. Personally, I believe that stress, fear, and anger are at the root of most diseases. Our bodies have a phenomenal ability to fight off germs, viruses, and bacteria, if we are not under the influence of stress; and since stress is only our perception of any given situation, we have the power to be stress-free.

Again, according to Levine:

> We face many choices in the course of a lifetime. We may not always be able to choose our circumstances, but we have the freedom to choose how we feel about those circumstances.
>
> Disease arises not so much out of what happens to us, but as a result of how we see things, and the things we tell ourselves. It isn't what happens that bugs you, it's the things that you say in your head about what happens that makes all the machinery get messed up and leads to a variety of diseases.

Simply put: **You are what you think and say.** If you are dreading bankruptcy and continue to feed the emotion, guess what happens? If you are jealous and fear that your significant other will cheat on you, guess what? If you are worrying about your health and fail to act, guess what?

EGO IS THE LACK OF BEING IN GOD'S SPIRIT. WE GIVE IT MORE POWER BY PAYING ATTENTION TO IT.

There are many good books on this subject, all based on scriptures, but I highly

recommend, *Hung By The Tongue*, by Francis P. Martin and
The Tongue: The Creative Force by Charles Capps.

Perhaps more than any other fact we have discussed
so far, the thought that you are what you think and say,
has both a powerful positive and negative potential. It is
also a prime demonstration of how the Mind and Body
work in concert. The Mind speaks to us both rationally
and emotionally with words, pictures, or images, which
can translate into physical conditions in the body.

One of the things I learned early on is that man is a far
more emotional creature than a logical one. Often, emotions (feelings) are negative, owing to the neural wiring
we have been saddled with, which goes
back to earliest man and the "flight or
fight" mechanism. Though we no longer
need to fear an attack by some great burly

ANY NEGATIVE
THOUGHT IS
STINKIN' THINKIN'

wild beast, there are still things in our culture and environment that are truly dangerous; thus we retain some
emotions (fear) as a protection.

However, this same emotion, fear, accounts for a great
deal of disharmony in our lives. When we are verbally
abused by an angry boss, for instance, the flight or fight
emotion nearly always kicks in automatically. Our first
reaction is to attack in kind, to become angry and defen-
sive, when in reality, if we allowed ourselves a few
seconds to reflect on what we perceived as an attack, our
logic or rational thinking would catch up, and when
applied properly, could diffuse the situation and perhaps
even teach us something in the bargain.

As is the case with most people who contract a life threatening illness, one of my earliest reactions to my disease, was frustration. I have never been one to get angry. However, I was completely *emotionalized* (stressed) about my predicament. Once I began to conduct my research into the Spirit, Mind, Body, connection, I began to learn how to change my thinking. I learned to turn the frustration and aggravation into logical, useful solutions. My original discouragement just fired me up to find answers. If Great-grandmother Soffe could walk barefoot from Iowa to Salt Lake City, I could certainly beat Parkinson's!

In another Chopra book, *The Seven Spiritual Laws of Success*, his first law, The Law of Pure Potentiality, states:

> *This law is based on the fact that we are, in our essential state, pure consciousness. Pure consciousness is pure potentiality; it is the field of all possibilities and infinite creativity . . .*
>
> *. . . This is our essential nature. When you discover your essential nature and know who you really are, in that knowing itself is the ability to fulfill any dream you have because you are the eternal possibility, the immeasurable potential of all that was, is, and will be.*
>
> *This law could also be called The Law of Unity because underlying the infinite diversity of life is the unity of one all-pervasive spirit. There is no separation between you and this field of energy. The field of pure potentiality is your own Self.*

And, the more you experience your true nature,
the closer you are to the field of pure potentiality.

In the perspective of this book, this potential would be the ability to heal yourself, or to avoid ever becoming ill in the first place.

Who are we? We are what we think and believe. Our minds are the most powerful force on earth. When I focused my mind on healing through daily meditation, prayer, and conscious thought, my life began to change. People often tell me that I'm a living prayer, meaning I'm constantly in a state of subtle meditation in the form of positive self-talk, prayer, and a very deliberate concentration on other people's well-being, not on myself.

I could go on for another 200 pages quoting the works of pioneers such as Dr. Candace Pert, Ph.D., Dr. Deepek Chopra, Barbara Hoberman Levine, Dr. Wayne Dyer, or Dr. Richard Gerber, among others, in the field of the Spirit, Mind, and Body connection. Suffice it to say, some reading in this area on your part will help you to more fully understand and accept the physical nature of these connections. (See Resource section in the back of this book.) Therefore, for the moment, let's just all agree to do one thing: keep an open mind. If only for the remainder of this book, try to suspend all your notions and biases regarding the medical establishment and the physical sciences. Instead, take a leap of faith with me and let us now look at the role that Spirit plays in all these connections.

The Spirit

Based on the examples I've just used, I think we can agree that at some point "belief" becomes "biology"; but where and how do belief, biology, and Spirit intersect, and how does that connection work?

"The Mind and Body Are One" From *The Power of Full Engagement*, by Jim Loehr and Tony Schwartz:

> *The primary markers of physical capacity are "strength, endurance, flexibility and resilience." These are precisely the same markers for our capacity for emotions, mentality, and spirituality. Flexibility at the physical level, for example, means that the muscle has a broad range of motion. Stretching increases flexibility.*
>
> *The same is true emotionally. Emotional flexibility reflects the capacity to move freely and appropriately along a wide spectrum of emotions rather than responding rigidly or defensively. Emotional resilience is the ability to bounce back from experiences of disappointment, frustration, and even loss.*
>
> *Mental endurance is a measure of the ability to sustain focus and concentration over time, while mental flexibility is marked by the capacity to move between the rational and the intuitive, and to embrace multiple points of view.*

> *Spiritual strength is reflected in the commit-*
> *ment to one's deepest values, regardless of*
> *circumstance and even when adhering to them*
> *involves personal sacrifice. Spiritual flexibility, by*
> *contrast, reflects the tolerance for values and*
> *beliefs that are different from one's own, so long as*
> *those values and beliefs don't bring harm to others.*
>
> *In short, to be fully engaged requires strength,*
> *endurance, flexibility,y and resilience in all the*
> *dimensions that are you.*

I had briefly mentioned before that we humans are endowed with awareness and free will, able to make choices and decisions. However, before awareness is trained, it is just energy and information. In order to change this energy into a usable form, we must train our minds to take on various tasks that are spiritual in nature. For example, in the case of my seemingly insurmountable "problem," I had to dig deep to find a spiritual solution. I had no choice. The doctors told me I would basically wither away and die. That was unacceptable to me. What did I do?

First, I realized that I had to bring all my energies together in balance. Without a clear and creative mind, I would not have been able to formulate our Parkimin Sprays. Without a spiritual connection, I would not have had the belief that a higher power was in control, and I would not have had the confidence to undergo my research. Without the proper diet and exercise, I would not have had the energy or clarity to even begin.

Secondly, I stopped focusing on the problem, as you and everyone else can. Reality only happened when I looked at it. *Did I want to see success or failure? What would I focus on,* I asked myself, *the life I want to live or the life I want to avoid?*

I then shifted my attention to my spiritual energy, which was not very difficult given my having been active in a spiritual environment most of my life.

You see, the energy of the Spirit is much stronger and faster than your physical energy or even the energy of your Mind, Body connection. The Spirit comes before the physical and mental aspects of our nature.

I decided immediately to turn the "problem" over to a higher power. In other words, I decided to **"let go"** and **"let God."** I realized that letting go has nothing to do with the release of anything outside of myself. The truth was that letting go was very simple and above all, natural. All living things are created to let go of the things that are not needed. It is important to know that *letting go* does not imply "surrender." It is asking God to take that burden from you so that you can go about the business of being creative, being alive and serving others, time far better spent.

> THERE IS NOTHING HIDDEN IN THE WORLD FROM THE MAN WHO WILL REVEAL HIMSELF, TO HIMSELF.
> —GUY FINLEY

Next, I began to view my surroundings and circumstances as forms of love rather than forms of fear. I then

reminded myself that I am an "infinite" soul in a temporary body and finally, through meditation and prayer, I
emptied my mind of all negativity.

*Last, I made a concerted effort to bring joy to every-
one around me as a means of eradicating my own
self-indulgence.*

All of this may sound simple, and it essentially is, but
like anything worthwhile it takes practice and I had nothing but time on my hands. It takes a daily diligence and
discipline, which some people think they do not have.

I try to be present and live in the now every waking
moment of each day and you can too. I wake up every
day with the very conscious intention to live that day in
a state of joy. Much of that comes from serving others
and not dwelling on negatives. I am also supremely
aware of what I say. I am careful to only say that which I
wish to create, which I want to come into existence.
Remember the old saying, "Be careful what you wish for,
you may get it"? I would modify that to read, "Be careful what you say, because you will create it. It will
manifest itself into your life."

When I first came to understand and know the world of
the Spirit, I could clearly see that all problems are illusions.
They are concocted by our infinitely creative minds (creativity has its good and bad sides). Many of us tend to
believe, through our creative thought, that we are separate
from our Source (in my case, I call that God), when in fact
we are not. We were all born perfect and about as close to
the Source as many of us will ever be again in our lifetimes.

Then, because we become conditioned by our parents, friends, society, Church, and teachers to believe that disease, premature aging, and stress are inevitable, we stray from the Source. But hear me now and hear me loud, **nothing comes into your life uninvited.** I knew that somehow I had invited this disease into my life subconsciously. I realized, like my grandfather had told me so many years before, "Billy, at my age, don't try to teach me, just *remind* me of what I agreed to do."

I needed to be reminded of something, but what? Oh, there were many: I needed to be reminded to bring joy into everyone's life. I needed to be reminded to *let go* and *let God*. I needed to be reminded to be present in every single moment of the day. I needed to remember that whatever I said or thought, I brought into creation. (In the book of Genesis in the Bible, it is written, "God spoke and the word was made flesh.")

This may sound odd but based on the way I live my life now, I consider that this disease was the best thing that ever happened to me. Not only am I more in love with life and everyone around me more than ever before, I was able to develop the Parkimin Sprays and a vital, healing protocol from which everyone can benefit.

We are our own worst enemies

Based on our conditioning, we all set up our own obstacles. We all come to believe that we do not have access to the Source and higher, faster forms of energy.

We come to believe that we are powerless in the face of the inevitable. Thus, from day one, we begin to die even as we grow. First, the Mind, Body connection begins to deteriorate and then the Spirit, Mind, and Body connection begins to disintegrate. It all becomes a self-fulfilling prophecy because the outcome is negativity, illness, and death. Society, the media, the medical establishment, and the drug companies bombard us with negative messages daily.

It does not have to work this way and in my case, it no longer does. What I came to understand in my deep reflections is that there is a universal intelligence at work (if you prefer to use this language instead of the words God or Spirit, and it is not my intention to foist "religion" or my spiritual beliefs on you, only that you trust in a power greater than yourself.)

It is a known scientific fact that every particle of matter, whether it be a constellation, mountain, or human being, responds to a message. This intelligence can be verified. We observe scientific laws as simple as gravity or as complex as quantum mechanics every day, and we never see *them*. When you eat a French fry, you don't think about how your body is going to turn that into new cells, or how it will go to replace the cells that make up the cornea of your eye. Universal Intelligence does that for you.

In his book, *There's a Spiritual Solution to Every Problem*, Dr. Wayne Dyer says:

You can literally rid yourself of any and all problems by seeing and implementing spiritual solutions.

Everything in our universe is nothing more than energy. That is, at the very core of its being, everything is vibrating to a certain frequency.

Slower frequencies appear more solid and this is where our problems show up. Faster frequencies such as light and thought are less visible. The fastest frequencies are what I call Spirit.

When the highest/fastest frequencies of Spirit are brought to the presence of lower/slower frequencies, they nullify and dissipate those things we call problems.

You have the power to increase your energy and access the highest/fastest energies for the purpose of eradicating any problems in your life.

Ultimately, it is your choice whether to align yourself with a high-energy field or a low one.

What he and others are saying is that accessing the Spirit is actually as simple as aligning yourself with the universal intelligence that is all about you, through the laws of physics.

In essence, all of nature exhibits a design to become its unique potential. All matter responds to a set of laws. One thing is certain: The deeper we probe the cosmos and the world of subatomic particles, the greater is our conviction that, with all the apparent chaos, AN ORDER

DOES EXIST. There is a tying together of all matter, an intelligent force binding, blending and emerging—a connection between you and every other human being, plant and animal and a connection between your SPIRIT, MIND, and BODY.

Dr. Carolyn Myss has devoted her work to what is referred to as "energy medicine." According to Myss, all humans are born with a body comprised of pure energy. She has studied the role of this energy as a healing agent. According to Myss, we can harness and direct this energy in amazing ways. (A list of her books and tapes in Resource section in the back of this book.)

Another great resource that involves our energy systems is the use of sound. At the Center for Neuroacoustic Research in Carlsbad, California, researchers are studying the matrix and boundaries of the physical, emotional, mental, and spiritual bodies through clinical and scientific research utilizing sound. According to their researchers, everyone has a "sound print" much like a fingerprint. Each of us has a fundamental tone, which resonates throughout (frequencies, not unlike brain wave frequencies) our body systems. Like the neurological and chemical reactions that take place within your body when you are fearful, the disruption of this tone or frequency that is unique to each of us, becomes disrupted when we are stressed, ill, angry, and fearful, or indulge in any negative emotions. I urge you to visit their Web site at: www.neuroacoustic.com. You will be amazed at what you learn and the documented results that they are getting. You will also find other very valuable links to everything we are discussing on our Web site at www.noparkinsons.net .

We can and do interfere with our brain's frequencies, our body's frequencies, and the chemical make up of our systems by our own actions, either consciously or subconsciously. We can interfere so much that our body's natural resistance to atrophy is negated. The result is that we begin to break down and become diseased. Our thoughts become disorganized and our connection to a higher power is severed or distorted.

The practical application of this powerful concept is that all we need to do is be *aware* that our lives are designed to exist in a state of incredible organization and then **trust that awareness** and use it to, among other things, affect a letting go of all our negative baggage. It is our desire to be in *control* of everything, *which is one of our strongest enemies.*

> SOUND BITES OF SOUND ADVICE, PROVIDE A SOUND FOUNDATION FOR HEALING.

We were all designed to express unimaginable potential and to interact with the matrix of life. We are all a part of the process designed to expand and become greater than we are individually. We were made to adapt and create by changing and becoming. All of our aspirations and dreams are potentialities waiting to be expressed into existence. In reality, all of nature is ready to assist us.

At some point, I had an epiphany. I was fully aware that for me to succeed, I had to accept that there was something at work for good in my life that was beyond my understanding. That is when I learned to let go.

Balancing Spirit, Mind, and Body

All of life is a balancing act and in today's hectic world, even if you're "healthy," your rhythms are often rushed, with your days being carved up into bits and bytes. Today's world tends to push us through our lives and we end up not really knowing who we want to be and where we are really going. Often, as was my case, stress and "dis-ease" are the ultimate outcome.

Like most everything in life, however, there is always a positive aspect to each negative outcome. Oddly, Parkinson's was not only an insidious disease, it was the motivating factor in my finally balancing my life spiritually, emotionally, and physically.

> WE ARE LIVING ART, CREATED TO HANG ON, STAND UP, FOR BEAR, CONTINUE, AND ENCOURAGE EACH OTHER.
> —MAYA ANGELOU

Let's begin with the word "energy" because contrary to popular belief, energy, not time, is our most precious resource. Everything we do, from our interactions with colleagues, friends, and family to making important decisions, requires energy. Disease, among other things, robs us of that vital reserve.

Likewise, every one of our words, thoughts, emotions, and behaviors has an "energy" consequence. To fully live in the present, to be completely engaged in our world, we must be balanced physically and be emotionally connected. We must be focused mentally and spiritually to a purpose beyond our immediate self-interests.

I realized early on that I had to draw on all four sources of energy in order to beat my disease. Balance is not one-dimensional. Each form of energy affects the other. It is simplistic but important to note that the mind does not function well if you don't pay attention to your diet. An obvious example would be the ingestion of too much processed sugars and fats, which not only causes weight problems, but leads to coronary heart disease, diabetes, and a host of other illnesses.

A proper diet is essential to a clear mind. Likewise, a daily or weekly physical regimen is just as important; be that walking, running, biking, hiking, weight training, or a combination of several options. There have been thousands upon thousands of books written on these subjects, so none of this common sense should be a revelation to anyone reading this book.

Let's take a look at both forms of energy. Physical energy capacity is measured in terms of quantity from low to high; emotional capacity is measured in terms of quality—negative or positive. These are our fundamental sources of energy. Let's call these the fuel that propels us on our daily mission.

If we practice and train our minds, and our bodies, it is possible to slow our decline physically and mentally, and actually deepen our emotional and spiritual capacity until the very end of our lives. It is also possible to eliminate stress and all disease and to ultimately lead lives of optimal well-being. But how do we begin?

The key to *balance* is to manage our energy, which means expending all three energies and then allowing ourselves, as top-notch athletes do, to renew.

The process of change

In my own daily regimen, I realized I had to make a drastic change in the way I was living. That became a three-step process that I call: **intention, reality**, and **action** (IRA).

First, I had to define my purpose, or intention. I had to break from the status quo and my habitual behaviors. I needed inspiration to do this, so I called on God through prayer and continual meditations. I wanted Him to help me spend my energy in ways that were consistent with my deepest values, which He did.

Understanding my own values fueled a compelling vision.

I got these from my family, friends, Church, coaches and teachers.

Next, I had to face reality, the truth. I knew I wasn't going anywhere until I could honestly identify who I truly was in my totality. Most of us regularly fool ourselves. We all want to avoid the unpleasant and discomforting things in our lives. In addition, we regularly underestimate the consequences of our energy management choices, which means failing to face up to what we're eating; how much exercise we're truly getting; how much mind power we are expending; how much energy we're investing in our family, friends, and work colleagues; and how often we have a dialogue with our Creator.

It was time for a reality check.

Finally, the third step, **action,** became a process of who I was and who I wanted to be. This became a blueprint for how I wanted to manage all my energies. As I said earlier, I begin every day with the intention of bringing joy into the world. In other words, I show up for life filled with positive energy every moment.

Now we are at the point in my story where I share my protocol. Of course, I use the Parkimin Sprays throughout the day, usually about six times. These sprays include the following, but are not limited to:

Co-enzyme Q-10, an important nutrient for the heart
Vitamins C, E, D, B-6, B-1, B-3, B-12
L-Dopa (Levadopa) which is a naturally occurring amino acid that converts into Dopamine and is used extensively with Parkinson's patients
GABA, a potent message-altering neurotransmitter, and many more too numerous to list here.

My protocol also includes my physical and diet regimen. Here is what my plan includes:

PROTOCOL FOR WILLIAM P. HANSEN

Spirit

Reading and listening to tapes daily. I particularly enjoy these authors:
- Wayne Dyer, Ph.D., *There is a Spiritual Solution to Every Problem,*
- Caroline Myss, Ph.D., *Sacred Contracts,* "By discovering your own spiritual energy and becoming aware of the lens through which

you see your world, you can change your mind and change your life."

- Richard Gerber, M.D., *Exploring Vibrational Medicine*

Mind

Once again, reading and listening to tapes helps me get my mind on the right path for the entire day. These inspirational tapes and books to remove "stinkin' thinkin'."

- Wayne Dyer, Ph.D.: *You'll See It When You Believe It*
- Depak Chopra, M.D.: *Ageless Body/Timeless Mind*
- Louise L. Hay: *The Power Within*
- Neale Donald Walsh: *Conversations with God*
- Caroline Myss, Ph.D.: *Why People Don't Heal*
- Norman Shealy, M.D. (and Caroline Myss): *The Creation of Health*

Body

I use Parkimin sprays throughout the day. My workouts consist of:

- Thirty minute workout with trainer three times a week for the first year (after first year on my own)
- Two mile walk or stationary bike three times a week
- Dancing two to three times a week

- Bottled water, 50 percent of body weight in ounces/day (suggest Penta™ water from Bio Hydration™)

BILL'S PROTOCOL
As of MAY 5, 2004

Cancer Protocol

- Natural Prostate Formula from Life Extension – two per day (has Saw Palmetto and other natural ingredients
- Lycopene (15mg) – two per day
- Resveratrol Caps, dietary supplement from Life Extension – two per day
- Boron, dietary supplement – two per day
- 4 injections of Lupron Depot. None in the last three months

All pills and capsules are purchased from
the Life Extension Foundation

Parkimin Sprays Protocol Nutrients

- Co-Enzyme Q10 – 1200ml per day
- Vitamin D3, 1000IU – one capsule per day
- Super Curcumin with bioperine, 900mg – two per day
- Super Zeaxanthin (5mg) with lutein (10mg) – one capsule per day
- Spray Technology (three sprays, three times per day)
  - Super Re-vital-izer (B Complex) from Parkimin Technologies
  - Spray-Eeze with Echinacea from Parkimin Technologies

- DHEA from Parkimin Technologies
- Memory Spray from Parkimin
  Technologies
- MSM and Ionics
- Parkimin Plus (six sprays, six times a day),
  twenty-two ingredients, L-glutathione – 300
  milligrams(approximate)
- Liquid ionic trace minerals – as directed by
  your nutrionist
- Fish Oil (Omega 3 and 6) by Carlson – two
  tablespoons (30ml) per day
- 1/3 cup of Flaxseed ground
- Vitamin C – 5000mg per day

An excellent resource for Spirit, Mind, and Body, protocol is Dr. Andrew Weil, author of *8 Weeks To Optimum Health, A Proven Program for Taking Full Advantage of Your Body's Natural Healing Power.*

Now, let's take a look at my protocol in more depth and what each area can bring to your life, too.

Body — Exercise

"Move it or lose it," is a familiar phrase to most of us. It applies to the exercise of the brain and mind itself as well as the body. Let's talk a little about what actually transpires within you (mind and body) when you engage in a weekly regimen of exercise.

Science and medicine have published countless research papers on the subject of exercise and its effect on the body as well as the mind. The simple movement of muscles (lifting your arms) stimulates the growth of axons, the appendage neurons that transmit impulses away from the cell body. These are the messages that go to other parts of the brain and to your body. Movement translates to more axons, which in turn is directly related to level of intelligence.

To my way of thinking, any life-altering changes in your Spirit, Mind, and/or Body must begin in your Mind as a desire to *change*. You will then need the fuel and the endurance (energy) to begin to make those profound changes in all of the parts that are you—your mind will have to be clear.

This is one of those proverbial chicken or egg paradoxes. Which comes first, the intention to change, or the physical exercise, which clears the mind enough to create the thought of intention in the first place? For our purposes, it doesn't matter. Do both simultaneously. The main point is to BEGIN. For the purposes of your program that by getting this far in the book, I assume you've already mentally and emotionally decided to change. At the end of this book, you will read about our Butt-n-Gear club. For now, understand the following thoughts are for you while you start your healing journey:

Are you ready to arrive? If so then do it now and get your "Butt-n-Gear." These are your ideal behaviors:

- *Repeated thanks to God for maintaining our passion to serve with hourly thanksgiving*

- *Out loud speaking into existence that which we visibly see or imagine.*
- *Constantly feeling with every power of spirit and mind, the magnificent result of helping people to a happy and productive life.*
- *What resources are required? New knowledge, clinical trials of the Parkimin Sprays, skillful associates dedicated to healing of Parkinson's and other related diseases and an attitude of progressive joy.*

Your exercise plan should include weights (even light hand weights are great), stretching, and walking, aerobic activity is also very important. The term "aerobic" literally means "with air," which means it's important to "challenge" your breathing. When you engage in aerobic exercise, you are actually growing new blood vessels and nerve cells (as well as growing axons in the brain). More blood vessels means more blood to the brain and the rest of your organs as well. It's that simple.

In addition, there are so many other benefits to aerobics. According to proven scientific studies, aerobic activity clearly improves the speed and quantity of memory recall, so important in many neurological disorders. It releases endorphins (those feel-good hormones) into your bloodstream, which allow us to relax and increase our cortical awareness (many of my best ideas come to me after riding the stationary bicycle fairly intensely for five minutes or more, and then I sprint for the last minute).

Aerobic exercise increases nerve growth agents. It builds optimism, so you are less likely to become depressed. It also does wonders for low self-esteem. When you begin to feel and look better to yourself, you act with far more confidence in everything that you undertake.

What could be a more positive motivator than knowing that as you exercise, you become more *intelligent*, more able to cope with stress, and more pleasant to be around?

Please see the Resource section in the back of this book for more specific programs that you can tailor to your own life-style. Know this, however: No matter what condition you're in or what age you are, there is an exercise program that can benefit you greatly. Any exercise is better than none. In a moment, I'll give you a brief description of what I do at the age of seventy-four. It's fairly rigorous, given my age, but if I can do it, you can too.

Contrary to popular opinion, walking is a fabulous exercise that almost everyone can do. Even when I had tremors and my motor skills were impaired early in my diagnosis, I walked.

Small hand weights are also helpful and relatively easy to work with for ten minutes, two or three times a day.

Stretching is vital as well. You should engage in light stretching prior to any aerobics and then as you begin to warm up, you can engage in stretches that are more strenuous. Use of a stationary bicycle is easy (they don't take up much room, or you can use the equipment in your community center, join a club or hire a trainer).

To my way of thinking, the key is to keep moving. I try walking instead of driving whenever possible. I never was a sedentary person, always prone to working in the garden, riding a bike, walking and, of course, dancing, (though at the time of this writing, a bone spur has greatly reduced my walking, but only temporarily). Swimming is also an excellent form of exercise.

Unfortunately, we are a nation of couch potatoes. Most of us sit through the day, either at work or at home, and we drive to nearly all our destinations, even the short ones.

Thousands of years ago, Paleolithic man was the picture of health. His lifestyle required him to hunt and to gather, nearly two-thirds of his day. There were no cases of hyperinsulinemia or high triglycerides. His body density was in perfect balance between fat and muscle. He was most decidedly a lean machine. He did, of course, succumb to various viruses and bacteria and, of course, was prey for larger, faster animals. The point is, Paleolithic man's simple diet and constant form of exercise was perfect for his environment and needs and there is no evidence that he ever suffered from Parkinson's, cancer, or any neurological disorders.

We have become sedentary through a combination of factors, including modern day society and the time constraints it foists upon all of us. But consider this: If you discovered one day that you had Parkinson's, would you have the time to address that issue and do something proactive about it? If you believe as I and millions of others do, that exercise could play a vital role in your healing process, would you find the time? Of course you would!

Finally, if you aren't currently active on a daily or at least weekly basis, you may find the change to a concerted exercise regimen stressful. Much the same also applies to your diet. The mind perceives "change" as a stressor. We are all much more comfortable with the status quo, particularly if things are going quite well. Therefore, as a stressor, a change in your lifestyle (eating habits and exercise) isn't always easy. It is important that you ramp up your mental and physical powers and accept that change is inevitable, particularly if you're suffering from a neurological disorder. You really have no other options. Be aware that what you are about to undertake will cause you some discomfort (stress) and perhaps even a little muscle pain, in the beginning. But, as with just about everything else in life, the journey of a thousand steps starts with one. Every step after that is easier and more delightful. It won't be long before you will thoroughly enjoy your personalized regimen and it won't be long before you'll wonder how you lived without it.

> EVERYTHING IN THE UNIVERSE HAS A RHYTHM. EVERYTHING DANCES.
>
> —MAYA ANGELOU

A final note: I think it's important to engage in the kinds of exercise that you enjoy. If you're like me and you like to . . . start dancing again. Perhaps you like a more competitive sport to keep your mind engaged; then play light competitive games in the beginning. My neighbor is an avid tennis player. He needs to do little else because in playing he not only stretches and builds muscle, he builds extremely high aerobic endurance. So, think tennis, lawn bowling, riding a bike, squash . . . whatever makes you happy.

Since my mind was unaffected by my Parkinson's, with the possible exception of a mild bout of depression now and again (I was lucky, most people with Parkinson's suffer debilitating forms of depression), I used my mind to access my spirituality and eventually formulate an exercise and diet plan to balance me in total.

The most important part of my diet was the use of our Parkimin Sprays, which provide the essential nutrients, amino acids, vitamins and other elements that enhance glutathione, which then converts to Dopamine.

Another side benefit of the sprays is their long shelf life. The glutathione that is injected (see earlier mention of Dr. Perlmutter's work), only has a forty-day shelf life. The Parkimin Sprays will stay fresh for four months because they use nitrogen to flush out all of the oxygen in the bottles.

Second, I hired a physical trainer and began a three-times-a-week, workout program. At first, of course, these were very mild as I had very little strength. Gradually, as I became more balanced mentally, emotionally, and spiritually, they became increasingly intense. (Confidence begets confidence.)

There was a two-mile walk (temporarily out of commission because of a bone spur in my foot), plus a fifteen-minute workout on the stationary bike with the last minute spent sprinting, and six minutes using an elliptical cross trainer.

My favorite form of exercise was my dancing, which I do with great enthusiasm two or three times every week. In order to make it easier for you to develop an exercise regimen and stick to it, I recommend your plan begin with something you love to do.

Here is a quote from my trainer:

> *Spirit, Mind, and Body are what Bill preaches. I have been training Bill for more than a year and a half. The fact that he has Parkinson's made me question how far his training would go. Our goals were for him to gain muscle, lose a small amount of body fat, and gain some strength.*
>
> *With Bill's consistent workouts and spray nutritionals (Body), positive attitude (Mind), and his early morning quiet time (Spirit), he has far exceeded my expectations. He has gained muscle and lost body fat. He is still gaining weight on the scale by dropping his body fat percentages. His tremors have diminished. But the greater improvement is how his strength has progressed. He is lifting more and more weight weekly. I almost can't believe it even though I see it.*
>
> *Bill truly is an inspiration, and all should follow his example. We would live healthier lives.*
>
> — Heather Young, AFFA
>   Trainer Fitness/Counselor
>   Carlsbad, California

Spirit Regimen

I meditate in the morning and afternoon. In addition, I indulge in several two to five minute "Wonder Sessions." We've all heard the old adage "Stop and smell the roses." Well essentially that's what a Wonder Session is. These can be walks on the beach, in a favorite park or along a special trail. When possible, I like to go barefoot and feel the grass or sand between my toes (park or beach). I breathe in the beauty and serenity that is all around me and remind myself how thankful I am (we all should be) to be able to enjoy the beauty of God's creation. I observe flowers, birds, clouds, and the smells, and find myself aware of them all, while at the same time, almost being in a meditative trance.

My primary focus is on *Spirit* and the bringing of joy into other people's lives. I do this by exerting a conscious effort every moment to balance my ego. By balance, I mean I strive to eliminate the need to win. I endeavor to eliminate the *me*-first attitude that can creep into my consciousness. I strive to see the other person's point of view first; to walk a mile in his shoes.

If you consider this fact: Ego=fear, you can take on a whole new perspective on life. As soon as we are fearful about anything, be it real or perceived, ego begins to take over. It is what our brains strive for because that is how we have been wired for thousands of years. Survival comes first and in today's world, that doesn't have to mean surviving a physical attack. It could simply be someone insulting you. Put another way, there is a great deal of credence given to the concept of forgiveness. And, that is good. However, in a perfect world, if each of us had strong self-esteem and were able to keep our ego in check, there would be no need for forgiveness because we never would have been hurt. Only the ego is hurt when we are attacked.

When the ego is in balance, it is easy to bring joy into other people's lives, because we are outwardly focused, not dwelling inwardly.

I wake up with this intention every day; to bring joy to others. To do that, I must balance my ego and be fully aware of those around me. And only when I am living in the moment can I have that awareness of the needs of others. People tell me that I have gotten to the point that I am a living prayer and that affirmation is that "thy will be done."

> ALL BEINGS HAVE THE CAPACITY TO CURE THEMSELVES.

I still read everything I can get my hands on, including re-reading all of the books in the Resource section of this book. Remember, we need to be reminded more than we need information. Therefore, we have designed our Web site to be interactive. We encourage an on-going dialogue so that your comments and input can encourage and inspire others.

Meditation

There are many forms of meditation. Prayer is one. There are also thousands of books written on this subject.

According to Dr. Frank Sovinsky, author of *Life: The Manual:*

> Basically, in order to heal any condition, the brain must get into a Delta and Theta brain wave for several hours a day. The dilemma is that we need to perform in the world, which is the Beta range, and it is also the brain wave that occurs when we are stressed. Thus, we need to make a great effort to think and not be controlled by the stress that emotions cause.
>
> You must essentially catch the perfect wave. Your brain has four frequencies (electrical impulses). Delta (.05–4Hz) is the longest and slowest wave needed for deep sleep and restoration. Theta (4–8Hz) is used for imaging and learning, plus a little daydreaming. When we are drifting in and out of sleep, we are in Theta. This state is difficult to maintain without practice, (e.g., a deep meditative state).
>
> Alpha (8–14Hz) is important in relaxation, visualization, daydreaming, and meditation. It is blocked by sensory awareness, conceptual thinking, and strong emotions.
>
> Beta (14–35Hz) is for action and task completion. It is the dominant wave when you are anxious, fearful, or alarmed.

We live our lives entering and exiting these energetic states. We shift from one to the other continuously during a day, depending upon the task at hand. If we are at ease, the brain is probably somewhere in the Alpha range. If anxiety is present, the brain shifts to higher Beta and it becomes necessary to find a way to guide it toward calmness and focus.

Awareness and the ability to alter these states puts you in charge of you! Learning is, in essence, a personal awakening, a realization that your thoughts influence the present and determine your future (you are what you think and say. Your ideas are essential to your well-being).

Our dilemma is this: You are a highly motivated individual. You have a drive to fulfill your purpose.

The challenge, if faced, is simple. Life is unpredictable and chaos is natural. It is our response to these events and processes that determines the outcome.

Every single day you experience 60,000 thoughts and process countless amounts of information. You awaken each morning with hopes of achieving great things, yet any strong visual, auditory, or kinesthetic distraction causes an internal fight or flight sympathetic reaction that distorts your perception and leads to poor judgment and performance.

Unfortunately, the brain does not have a filter to strain out all of the negative things, so this information is stored for permanent recall. And whether we like it or not, these emotional memories cloud our vision and limit our progress.

I couldn't agree more with the good doctor. Being aware of his observations from earlier research, I undertook biofeedback sessions with Lisa Tataryn. That was two years ago when I was still having serious prostate problems. As you might imagine, because of the prostate cancer and Parkinson's, my Beta waves were off the charts.

Although unable to return to Lisa for two years, I followed my protocol with practical determination, finally resuming my sessions with her last month. This is a note she sent to Scripps Institute with regard to my current status.

Re: Bill Hansen:

Parkinson's patients normally present with slowed Alpha (around 6–7 Hz). (Normal adults range from 9–13 HZ). Bill did not present with slowed Alpha. His Alpha brain wave was in the range of normal for his age group.

Two years ago, Bill's Alpha presented in the typical Parkinson's 6Hz but now, in 2004, his Alpha is at 8–9 Hz.

Sincerely,

Lisa Tataryn, B.Sc., R.P.C.C.N.P.

There are no signs of the previous wavelength patterns, and a visit to my urologist indicated my PSA levels are now normal.

The spirituality that gives me strength is not only derived from a lifetime of being blessed with incredibly strong, principled and loving mentors and friends, it is also derived from practicing daily meditation, or a conscious effort to put myself in Theta brainwave states.

Whether you choose deep breathing or some other relaxation technique (I use deep breathing and a mantra) to reach this state is up to you. I meditate three times daily for periods of about fifteen minutes each. My mantra is, "Thy will be done." Of course you can use any mantra you choose. Regardless of how you choose to get into this state, the point is to empty your mind of all thought, to make your mind vacant of all the clutter and static that Dr. Sovinsky mentioned. This exercise not only gives my body a deep rest, it fills me with creativity and inner strength.

> ALL STATES OF MIND REPRODUCE THEMSELVES.

This is all designed to focus my spiritual strength, and is reflected in the commitment to my deepest values, regardless of circumstance, and even when adhering to them involves personal sacrifice.

Mind

A writer friend of mine told me his mantra: "We only write as well as we think." This is true of any actions we undertake, whether they be writing, playing golf, or managing our energy.

I used inspirational tapes and books to remove what I call "Stinkin' Thinkin'," in particular the book I already mentioned, *Your Body Believes Every Word You Say*, by Barbara Hoberman Levine. Concisely, Levine indicates that, **"We are what we think and say."**

All those negative thoughts, even the ones you keep to yourself, affect you in profound ways. Positive begets a positive nature and negative begets a negative outcome. Essentially, you become what you say and think.

Of course, it was the proper management of my mind and emotional energy that led me to begin my work in researching the proper vitamin, amino acid, and other natural substances that ultimately became the Parkimin Sprays.

I also can't overstate the importance of participating in a support group. In Napolean Hill's historic work, *The Laws of Success*, he speaks about the **"Master Mind Theory,"** which essentially states that two heads are better than one and three are better than two. Hill postulates that when two or more minds work together, it is the equivalent of having another mind in the room, or a Master Mind.

In my Master Mind group of four people, we discuss our lives, exchange ideas and information, encourage each other and, of course, pray together. Each of us is striving to bring joy, peace, and understanding into the lives of the others.

Man is a social animal. His interdependence with others is a scientific fact. It becomes our common sense duty to become free, warm, loving, affirmative, social personalities and, thus, exercise our instinctive urge to give, to turn outward to others. The realization of the Spirit within you is dependent upon a sense of the "greater you," an ability to give, that can only be achieved by social interaction with others.

The power of humor

I also found that a sense of humor was imperative in my healing and the surest way to express this was to be socially active and share that outlook with others who, in turn, would share it with me. The word, "spirituel" (not spiritual) comes to mind here. The dictionary defines it thusly:

"spi•ri•tu•el or spi•ri•tu•elle - adj.
1. Of a refined and graceful mind or wit
2. light and airy in movement; ethereal

Generally, being *spirituel* is characterized by higher and finer things of the mind. It is a sense of balance, of the appropriateness and ridiculousness of things, of humility in self-love, of courage in faith.

Humor is a life preserver in a sea of gloom,
a vacuum cleaner for the unconscious, and an
element that preserves romance. It is prayer
in action, movement in contemplation. It pre-
vents fanaticism and dullness. It takes the

worm out of the apple of egotism and creates
a democracy among conflicting selves.

Humor is the gyroscope by which life can
be kept in balance between today and tomor-
row, between what is, and what can be,
between the conscious and the unconscious,
and between letting go and self-discipline.

— Fred Whitman

In addition, let's not forget that laughing stimulates the production of endorphins that sooth us and stimulate the immune system to great activity. Norman Cousins is known as the founder of psychoneuroimmunology. He literally laughed himself to good health and even used old Laurel and Hardy slapstick comedy tapes, and The Three Stooges tapes to lull himself to sleep. In his original studies, he called the ability to mentally influence the immune system with humor as "hardiness." His concepts included the critical ingredient of a positive attitude, which he defined as maintaining a sense of humor and general joyfulness. He called it "internal jogging." He discovered firsthand that laughter can help in the recovery from life-threatening illnesses and that even a few moments of laughter can reduce inflammation in the body.

He also found that these benefits were derived from laughter:
- Enhanced respiration
- An increased number of immune cells
- A decrease in cortisol (the chemical your
  body uses to prepare you for fight or flight)

- An increase in endorphins (that "feel good" hormone)
- An increase in salivary immunoglobulin type A concentrations

He also discovered that problem-solving abilities yield far better results when they are preceded by laughter, which has a way of turning off posterior hypothalamic activity and allowing the cerebral cortex to carry on stress-free activity.

Cousins' studies concluded that ten minutes of laugher can provide a person who is in pain with at least two hours of good sleep. He was also famous for creating a "humor cart" including comic books, comedy tapes, audiotapes, humorous books and magazines—all intended to induce laughter that many hospitals use today, especially in their oncology departments.

In short, give yourself permission to perform an entire range of laughs every day, from the simple social titter to the gut busting belly laugh, and you'll feel a lot better, whether you're sick or not.

Everyone responds to different types of laughter from a simple joke to slapstick pratfalls and everything in between. Start a humor file or box in your home. Fill it with funny tapes, books, magazines, jokes, or whatever amuses you. You can even go online to www.touchstarpro.com/smile-software.html and order your own personal humor profile software for just $9.95.

Lastly, do as I do and try to see the humor in everything around you. Life is filled with laughter. If you can laugh at yourself and the humor around you, you'll not only be a happier person, you'll be much healthier.

Diet

My eating habits are based on *The Zone Diet* and *The Omega Zone* by Dr. Barry Sears. In essence, the diet is quite simple. You have no doubt heard the saying that "The body is the temple for your mind." Throughout this section, I've been discussing the need to create a body within which your mind can thrive.

THE BEST DOCTORS IN THE WORLD ARE DR. DIET, DR. QUIET AND DR. MERRYMAN.
—JONATHON SWIFT

My diet became a complete way of life for me. Actually, I prefer the term "eating habits" as opposed to diet. To develop the energy levels I needed physically, I had to eliminate mostly refined sugars, processed complex carbohydrates and fats, preservatives, chemicals, and animal and plant byproducts.

I won't spend a great deal of time on this subject, because there is so much good material devoted to diet (see Resource section), however, it is important to note that there is a very close relationship between diet and the brain and mind. The connection between mind and diet is no less crucial than between mind and body.

The National Research Council, after reviewing more than 5,000 studies, published a 1,300-page report in 1989 entitled, *Diet and Health: The Implications for Reducing Chronic Disease Risk.* You can view these findings at www.usda.gov/fcs/cnpp online.

In general, the study found that Americans eat excessive amounts of fat, simple carbohydrates and too much refined sugar. This should come as no surprise given the dialogue in the media about fast food and obesity.

The study recommends many of the same things that are contained in The Omega Zone diet, including an emphasis on fish (Omega-3 fats), skinless poultry, lean meats, low-fat and non-fat dairy products and complex carbohydrates, which would include fruits and vegetables.

There is a raging debate in this country, not so much over the above-mentioned types of foods, but the quantity of each. A number of experts recommend your diet consist of 55 percent carbohydrates, 25 percent protein, and 20 percent to 25 percent non-saturated fats. The Omega Zone diet recommends a nearly even division of these components.

Each of us is different, so it is difficult to dictate what will work for you. A little common sense, however, goes a long way. If you are a very active person, you will need carbohydrates that are more complex in your diet; but I think we all agree (as a nation) that we could certainly use far less refined carbohydrates, sugars, and saturated fats in our diets.

A recent article in the *Los Angeles Times* spoke about Omega-3 fatty acids:

> *Behavior linked to consumption of fish oil*
> *February 2004*
>   *People who eat fish rich in heart-healthy Omega-3 fatty acids, such as salmon and tuna,*

*appear to have less hostility than those who don't
eat such fish.*

*Dr. Carlos Ibarren, a researcher with Kaiser
Permanente in Oakland, and colleagues at several
medical centers, analyzed eating habits and psychological tests of 3,581 urban adults, ages eighteen to
thirty, who participated in a federal heart study.
After the researchers adjusted for factors such as age,
sex, race, education, employment, smoking, drinking, and weight, they found that eating fish high in
Omega-3 fatty acids was an independent predictor
that someone would score lower on measurements of
hostility, including cynicism and mistrust of others,
anger, and aggression.*

*The findings, published in the January issue of
the European Journal of Clinical Nutrition, follow
Japanese research from 2000 that found fish oil supplements lowered aggression in students dealing
with the stresses of final exams, and a 1992 U.S.
study that found a cholesterol-lowering high-fish
diet reduced hostility and depression in adults.*

Wow! Looks like a heavy dose of fish, particularly
salmon and tuna, and a lot of laughing, can really pay off.

The important thing to consider and remember is that
whatever diet regimen you follow, failure to consume a
balanced diet will take its toll on brain function!

The Dancin' Again Club
I Did (have Parkinson's) But I Don't (now)
(IDBID)

Parkimin Technologies is dedicated to providing natural tools, including a program for educating the individual through the Spirit, Mind, and Body, for the control of Parkinson's and other neurological disorders.

To purchase the Parkimin Plus sprays we encourage you to go online now to **www.noparkinsons.net**. And follow the simple instructions on the **Spray Store** page.

To join this interactive club, go to **The Dancin' Again Club** page, where you will find special offers, timely insights on new discoveries, and up-to-the-minute alternative and complimentary treatments as well as a host of valuable links to other sites.

> WE NEED REMINDERS MORE THAN WE NEED KNOWLEDGE.

A monthly newsletter is available on the site as well. And we encourage you to share your experiences, comments, and insights with us.

Mostly, **The Dancin' Again Club** is a wonderful support mechanism. A friend of mine for many years always used an expression that I loved, "Get your butt in gear and get the job done," he always used to say. When you join the **Dancin' Again Club**, we'll send you a handy medallion/key chain that contains a tiny gear on which the inscription reads, "Butt-'n-Gear. Now you can get the job done." Reminders are more important than education.

The IDBID page is our way of helping you get your butt in gear, to take charge of your life through your natural Spirit, Mind, and Body connections.

I know the positive effects of a health support group firsthand. Several years ago I met a woman, Reverend Nancy Berggren, who has become a dear friend. She, in turn, introduced me to a woman in the Church, Esther Jones, who was starting a group. She called it her "Master Mind" group, after the concepts in Napoleon Hill's book. I began meeting with this group and immediately felt a sense of community and loving support that has gone a long way to help me in my healing process, so much so that we have patterned our Web site upon the principles of loving support.

Following is a letter written by Reverend Berggren.

> *Bill Hansen's dream is to eradicate Parkinson's disease globally, much as polio and smallpox were eliminated. A challenging but lofty dream to be sure, but my friend Bill may be just the one to help usher in such a remote possibility.*
>
> *I got to know Bill about two years ago, although we'd been introduced some time before. We began meeting weekly at 7:00 A.M. in a Master Mind group to support one another in realizing our dreams. When I heard Bill talk about his dream, and about how far he had come in his own rehabilitation, I was instantly enthralled.*

I have watched him battle through bouts of early morning tremors. I've watched him use himself as a guinea pig to prove or disprove each of the steps along the way of his "protocol;" going through his own private hell with reactions to different combinations of drugs, searching endlessly for an answer to help end the suffering of so many. He even invited me to go dancing one Thursday evening. I have been a professional dancer; I can tell you this man knows how to move on the dance floor!

The most devastating aspect of this disease, as he explains it, is that the doctors really can offer no hope to its suffering victims. Bill doesn't claim to have found a "cure" for Parkinson's, but from what I have seen with my own eyes, the hope his oral sprays offer will seem like nothing less than a miracle to those who currently have none.

I am grateful to know this man and to see the passion with which he has dedicated his life to alleviating the suffering of others. I joyfully give my permission to use any or all of this letter in any way to help speed the process of making his dreams a reality NOW!

Peace and Joy,
The Reverend Nancy Berggren
Senior Minister
First Church of Religious Science

The Reverend is an active member of **The Dancin'
Again Club** as is Lorraine Butler, who wrote this letter:

Dear Bill:

*I am finding that since I have taken your
Parkimin Plus spray product, I have nothing but
praise to share with you with regards to your product. In addition, how meaningful my physical and
emotional response has been. My feelings are very
deep and I don't know if I can find the words to
convey them. I'll just try to share where I was
physically and emotionally.*

*Sometimes there are events and occurrences
that come along in your life with enough impact to
literally change the course of your life and for me
this is one of those occurrences. Thank you, Bill
Hansen, for making this wonderful product a reality in my life. I would very much like to be a part
of sharing this information with all who need to
hear it.*

*Today I drove myself to the store. I did my own
grocery shopping. I wrote my own grocery list and
was able to read it. Now these are all simple things
and they may not sound like much in the ordinary
lives of everyone, but for me, they were absolutely
"perfect gifts." Parkinson's disease has challenged
me for more than fifteen years and for fourteen of
those, I was able to maintain myself quite well.
About a year ago, everything became much more difficult, a condition to which I had, for lack of a better*

word, "stabilized." Three months ago, however, I "unstabilized." My ability to walk became severely compromised. Driving was not comfortable for me and writing had become a thing of the past.

Bill Hansen, President of MJB Global, has just developed a product that I was fortunate enough to learn about and start using. Parkimin Plus is an absolutely amazing product. And, I will never be without it in my life again.

I have been using Parkimin Plus for eight straight days. My tremors are down by 90 percent! . . . rigidity about 90 percent gone! I am experiencing clarity of mind and thought and that is a joy. My speech is for the most part clear and without a slur. The continuous tremors are gone. Some sporadic ones do appear, but do not stay for any length of time. And, what I term as the "terrible tremors" have not appeared for days.

The clarity of thought for me means the words I want to use are more accessible to me. I am remembering more, forgetting less and my mind feels clear and sharp again. In addition, the ability to write has come back. I was finally able to write my grocery list . . . and to read it while shopping.

It is amazing when things start coming back to you that have been lost. It's as if they have never been gone.

Rigidity was especially difficult for me. The tremors are bad, but this rigidity is the one thing

that takes your life away and when that happens,
all the scary things happen. So many of us have a
tendency to take these little things for granted and
assume they will always be there . . . such as the
ability to walk, to swallow, or to move from a
seated or lying position. My ability to walk became
severely compromised almost overnight.

In any case, I am here to say that I'm well on the
road to recovery and am a very appreciative per-
son. Thank you and God bless you.

Sincerely,
Lorraine Butler

When you visit our Web site: www.noparkinsons.net, you will find many other beautiful testimonials, along with a wealth of other information.

In closing, don't forget to utilize the many resources listed on the following pages.

Meanwhile I wish all of you HOPE, love, and serenity. With all my love and encouragement.

Bill Hansen

Thy will be done.

The
Parkimin
Mission Statement

The fulfillment of a thirteen-year dream that Spray Technology will become *the* delivery system of choice for the world's nutritional needs.

Physicians will recognize that Absorption, Balance, and Stability (ABS) are the best keys to nutrition and mechanical delivery.

Master fulfillment of this dream is Parkimin Technologies, Inc. being the catalyst to bring about **HOPE** to all physically challenged people and further scientific solutions to the diseases that heretofore have had no cure.

List of Resources

Books (In random order)

Ageless Body Timeless Mind
Deepek Chopra, M.D.

The Seven Spiritual Laws of Success
Deepek Chopra, M.D.

Healing Myths Healing Magic
Donald M. Epstein

Molecules of Emotion
The Science Behind Mind-Body Medicine
Candace Pert, Ph.D

Your Body Believes Every Word You Say
Barbara Hoberman Levine

The Power of Full Engagement
Jim Loehr and Tony Schwartz

Conversations With God
Neale Donald Walsch

Climbing Higher
Montel Wlliams

The Secret of Letting Go
Guy Finley

Life: The Manual
Dr. Frank Sovinsky

The Owner's Manual-The Brain
Pierce J. Howard, Ph.D.

The Mind & The Brain
Neuroplasticity and the Power of Mental Force
Jeffrey M. Schwartz, M.D., and Sharon Begley

Hung By The Tongue
Francis P. Martin

Why God Won't Go Away
Brain Science and The Biology of Belief
Andrew Newberg, M.D.
Eugene D'aquili
Vince Rause

Exploring Vibrational Medicine
Richard Gerber, M.D.
(Books and tapes available through **Sounds True**, Carolyn Myss, Ph.D.)

The Anatomy of Hope
How People Prevail In The Face of Illness
Jerome Groopman, M.D.

8 Weeks To Optimum Health
A Proven Program for Taking Full Advantage of Your Body's Natural Healing Power.
Dr. Andrew Weil

100 Questions and Answers About Parkinson's
Abraham Lieberman, M.D.

The Omega RX Zone
The Miracle of the New High-Dose Fish Oil
Dr. Barry Sears

You Gotta Keep Dancin'
Tim Hansel

Thought as Energy
*Exploring the Spiritual
  Nature of Man*
Thelma Moss (And many
  others)

*You're Not Sick, You're
  Thirsty*
*Water for Health, for
  Healing, for Life*
F. Bateman Ghelidj, M.D.

The 12 Stages of Healing
Donald M. Epstein, D.C.

*Shaking Up Parkinson's
  Disease*
*Fighting Like A Tiger,
  Thinking Like A Fox*
Abraham Lieberman, M.D.

*The Complete
  Encyclopedia of
  Natural Healing*
Gary Null, Ph.D.

Let's Communicate
The American Parkinson
  Disease Association

The Cure For All Diseases
Hulda Regehr Clark,
  Ph.D., N.D.

PD "n" Me
The American Parkinson
  Disease Association

*Parkinson's Disease
  Handbook*
The American Parkinson
  Disease Association

Be Active
*A Suggested Program for
  People With Parkinson's
  Disease*
The American Parkinson
  Disease Association

*Patient Perspectives on
  Parkinson's*
Sid & Donna Dorros

*Water, The Foundation of
  Youth, Health and
  Beauty*
William D. Holloway, Jr. &
  Herb Joiner-Bey, N.D.

The Calcium Factor: The Scientific Secret of Health and Youth
Robert R. Barefoot & Carl J. Reich, M.D.

Love, Medicine & Miracles
Bernie S. Siegel, M.D.

The Complete System of Self-Healing (Internal Exercises)
Dr. Stephen T. Chang

Lucky Man
A Memoir
Michael J. Fox

Your Sacred Self
Making the Decision To Be Free
Dr. Wayne W. Dyer

You'll See It When You Believe It
Dr. Wayne W. Dyer

There's a Spiritual Solution to Every Problem
Dr. Wayne W. Dyer

The Clinician's Handbook of Natural Healing
Gary Null, Ph.D.

SynchroDestiny
Discover the Power of Meaningful Coincidence
Deepek Chopra, M.D.

Good Nutrition in Parkinson's Disease
The American Parkinson Disease Association

Meaning & Medicine
Larry Dossey, M.D.

Death By Diet
Robert R. Barefoot

The Sanctuary
The Path To Consciousness
Stephen Lew & Evan Slawson

Boom, You're Well
Douglas Hunt, M.D.

*Parkinson's Disease, A
   Complete Guide for
   Patients & Families*
William J. Weinger, M.D.
Lisa M. Shulman, M.D.

*Dr. Wright's Little Book of
   Big Health Secrets,
   Vols. I & II*
Dr. Jonathan Wright

*Understanding
   Parkinson's Disease*
GlaxoSmithKline

*The Parkinson's
   Handbook*
Dwight C. McGoon, MD

HELPFUL PHONE NUMBERS

American Healthcare Association
(202) 842-4444

Americans With Disabilities Act
Regional & Technical Assistance Centers
(800) 949-4232

National Council On Aging
(202) 479-1200

Elder Care Information & Referral Service
(800) 677-1116

IMPORTANT WEB SITES

The Dancin' Again club
Hope Heals
   www.noparkinsons.net

We Move
   www.wemove.org

The National Parkinson Foundation, Inc.
   www.parkinson.org
American Parkinson Disease Association
   www.apdaparkinson.com

Lisa Tataryn (Bio-feedback)
   www.nfcenter.com

For humor:
   www.touchstarpro.com/smile-software.html

The Center for Neuroacoustic Research
   www.neuroacoustic.com

Powerful Therapy for Challenging Brain Disorders
David Perlmutter, MD
   Brain Recovery.com

More Web Sites

   www.onhealth.com

   www.webmd.com

   www.aolhealth.com

   www.drkoop.com

   www.healtheon.com

   www.ama.com

   www.betterhealth.com

   www.healthanswers.com

   www.lhealthatoz.com

   www.mayohealth.org

www.healthconnect.com

www.medscape.com

www.healthgate.com

www.mediconsult.com